Herbal Remedies for Sleep

HOW TO USE HEALING HERBS AND NATURAL THERAPIES to Ease Stress, Promote Relaxation, and Encourage Healthy Sleep Habits

Maria Noël Groves

Storey Publishing

The mission of Storey Publishing is to serve our customers by
publishing practical information that encourages
personal independence in harmony with the environment.

EDITED BY Carleen Madigan
ART DIRECTION AND BOOK DESIGN BY Bredna Lago
TEXT PRODUCTION BY Jennifer Jepson Smith

COVER PHOTOGRAPHY BY © Alain Jarrad/Shutterstock, front t.c.; © AmyLv/Shutterstock, front small white flowers; © azure1/Shutterstock, front 2nd fr. b.c., t.c.r.; © FotoHelin/Shutterstock, spine; © Gummy Bear/Shutterstock, front 2nd fr. b.l., 2nd fr. b.r.; © haraldmuc/Shutterstock, front m.r.; © HHelene/Shutterstock, front b.c.; © Ilizia/Shutterstock, front t.l.; © Jay Gao/Shutterstock, front b.r.; © New Africa/Shutterstock, front 3rd fr. b.l.; © oksana2010/Shutterstock, front b.l.; © Spalnic/Shutterstock, front m.l., b.c.r.; © Stacey Cramp, back (all ex. bckgd.), front 3rd fr. t.l., 4th fr. b.r.; © Svetlana Zhukova/Shutterstock, front t.r.; © Swisty242/Shutterstock, front 2nd fr. t.r.; © Vit_Os/Shutterstock, front 2nd fr. t.l., 3rd fr. b.r.; © Vitek Prchal/Shutterstock, front and back, bckgrd.

INTERIOR PHOTOGRAPHY BY © Stacey Cramp
ADDITIONAL PHOTOGRAPHY BY © 1168group/Shutterstock, 3; © ADVTP/Shutterstock, 44 l.; © Alain Jarrad/Shutterstock, 87; © Alena Ozerova/Shutterstock, 9; © alexmak7/Shutterstock, 44 r.; © Alice Arts Bar/Shutterstock, 122 and throughout (background); © AmyLv/Shutterstock, iv white flowers; © Artem Avetisyan/Shutterstock, 162; © azure1/Shutterstock, 85; © B Lamb/Shutterstock, 22; © Bapi Ray/Shutterstock, 12 l.; © Chase D'animulls/Shutterstock, 94; © djgis/Shutterstock, 78; © Dudakova Elena/Shutterstock, 65; © Flas100/Shutterstock, 5 background (and throughout); © FotoHelin/Shutterstock, 92; © Grigorev Mikhail/Shutterstock, 18; © Gummy Bear/Shutterstock, v b.c.; © Heike Rau/Shutterstock, 21 b.r.; © HHelene/Shutterstock, 98; © Ilizia/Shutterstock, 62; © Image Source/Alamy Stock Photo, 25; © Indian Food Images/Shutterstock, 30; © JIANG TIAN-MU/Shutterstock, 15 r.; © John Polak, 141; © Julia Ardaran/Shutterstock, 41; © Kabar/Shutterstock, 15 l., 74 l.; © Kseniia Perminova/Shutterstock, 75 r.; © Lisa A/Shutterstock, 159; © littlenySTOCK/Shutterstock, 46; © Luria/Shutterstock, 159 (background); © Manfred Ruckszio/Alamy Stock Photo, 71; Courtesy of Maria Noël Groves, 21 l., 68; © meeboonstudio/Shutterstock, 104; © Musat/iStock.com, 61; © Nadezhda Kulikova/Shutterstock, viii; © Neil Lockhart/Shutterstock, 81; © New Africa/Shutterstock, iv pink flowers; © oksana2010/Shutterstock, 91; © Olechka K/Shutterstock, 40; Pauline Jurkevicius/Unsplash, 88; © Steffen Hauser/botanikfoto/Alamy Stock Photo, 73; © Strelyuk/Shutterstock, 12 r.; © Sundry Photography/Shutterstock, 90; © tarapong srichaiyos/Shutterstock, 29 l.; © Tatyana Soares/Shutterstock, 10; © Uros Poteko/Alamy Stock Photo, 77; © Vaclav Mach/Shutterstock, 17 l., 100; © Varts/Shutterstock, 53; Vero Manrique/Unsplash, 26; © VH-studio/Shutterstock, 21 t.r.; © Vit_Os/Shutterstock, v t.r.; © wasanajai/Shutterstock, 43, 75 l.; © Zula Albab/Shutterstock, 76 r.

TEXT © 2024 by Maria Noël Groves

Storey books may be purchased in bulk for business, educational, or promotional use. Special editions or book excerpts can also be created to specification. For details, please contact your local bookseller or the Hachette Book Group Special Markets Department at special.markets@hbgusa.com.

Storey Publishing
210 MASS MoCA Way
North Adams, MA 01247
storey.com

Storey Publishing is an imprint of Workman Publishing, a division of Hachette Book Group, Inc., 1290 Avenue of the Americas, New York, NY 10104. The Storey Publishing name and logo are registered trademarks of Hachette Book Group, Inc.

ISBNs: 978-1-63586-774-9 (paperback); 978-1-63586-783-1 (ebook)

Printed in the United States by Versa Press on paper from responsible sources
10 9 8 7 6 5 4 3 2 1

Library of Congress Cataloging-in-Publication Data on file

GRATITUDE AND ACKNOWLEDGMENTS

No herbalist comes into being without the teachings and shared experiences of others. My deepest gratitude to everyone who has contributed to the body of knowledge represented in this book. This includes my primary herb teachers Michael Moore, Rosemary Gladstar, Nancy and Michael Phillips, and Christine Tolf, as well as David Winston, Mary Bove, Rosalee de la Forêt, Aviva Romm, Thomas Easley, Tori Hudson, and Daniel Gagnon, among many others including the Indigenous peoples of the world, upon whose traditions modern herbalism is founded. I've perused and appreciated access to a world of scientific literature freely available via PubMed and GoogleScholar, as well as the robust and even-keeled safety data in the AHPA's *Botanical Safety Handbook*. Thank you, especially, to the students, clients, and others who have shared their experiences with the plants with me and helped me better understand the nuances of the plants and how individual people interact with them. The plants themselves, and our experiences with them, are our best teachers. So many people have found these plants to be important allies in their personal journeys to better sleep, relaxation, and mood, including me.

Contents

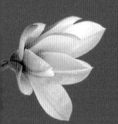

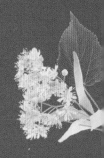

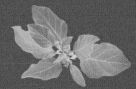

My Story of Sleep

My own journey into herbalism began with sleep and the herbs you'll learn about in this book.

After a traumatic set of events during my sophomore year of college, I found myself overcome by panic attacks and insomnia for months. I had a racing heart, nightmares, and an incessant buzzing sensation throughout my body that made me feel like I'd just gulped a gallon of coffee. I didn't know it at the time, but my body was stuck in fight-or-flight mode. It prevented quality sleep, and that lack of sleep fueled the vicious cycles of PTSD, stress, anxiety, and insomnia.

I've probably always been on the uptight side. I've needed more hours of sleep to maintain well-being than most people do, from the moment I emerged from the womb. Throughout my life, if I didn't get my sleep, my mood and health (and therefore the mood and health of those around me) immediately suffered. My mother dreaded my sleep-deprived return from childhood slumber parties. Even though my own life has been blessed, I've inherited trauma from past generations that has permeated and easily disrupts the balance of many in my extended family. But this was my first time experiencing such a degree and duration of anxiety and insomnia.

Fortunately, I'd also just begun reading about herbal medicine. Eventually it dawned on me that maybe herbs could help. I walked into the local herb shop and asked the staff for guidance. They pointed me toward tinctures of kava for the anxiety and valerian for sleep—two of the most popular herbs in the renaissance of herbalism in the late 1990s. Until that point, my limited understanding of herbs came from a few books and magazine articles. I hadn't *experienced* the herbs. The moment I took the tinctures, I noticed a downregulation of the panic that had been flooding my body. My sleep wasn't perfect, but it was better. I also did a lot of deep work to address my trauma and fear, but the herbs helped make it possible.

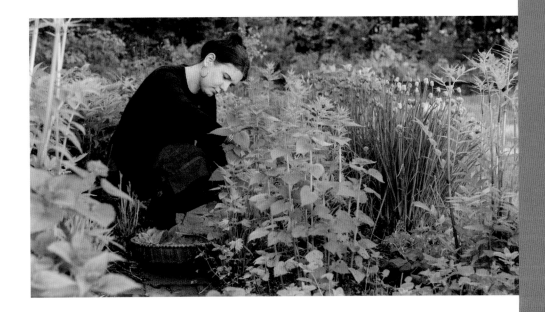

From that moment forward, herbs became the centerpiece of my life. When I graduated with my journalism degree, I went to work as an editor for *Natural Health* magazine, covering the herb beat and running the fact-checking department. I interviewed some of our most revered herbalists across the country, learned how to read scientific literature, and slowly built my herbal library. Eventually it became clear that I needed to do more, and I spent the next years moving from one herbal program to another, to work toward a career as an herbalist. I ultimately began teaching and seeing clients. Flash forward several decades later, and I am honored and grateful to have connected with a community of people and plants centered on healing.

The plants have an amazing capacity not only to help us feel better in the moment but also to shift our outlook on the world. Perhaps you're new on this journey and are struggling with sleep and anxiety; you're certainly not alone. Maybe you're just hoping that one remedy from this book will help you sleep better. I hope you'll find that in these pages, but I suspect you've also begun a deeper journey into the world of herbs that will enrich your life in ways you never knew possible.

—Maria Noël Groves

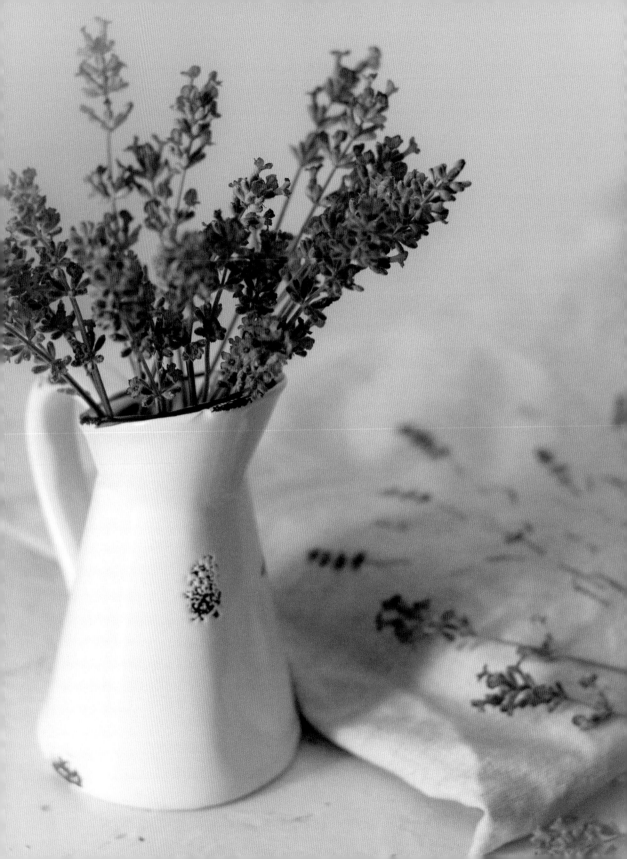

CHAPTER 1

Understanding and Supporting Quality Sleep

Sleep is a foundational aspect of our health and well-being. With sleep, the body functions well. When sleep is shortchanged or disrupted, we feel it on multiple levels both immediately and over the long term. Herbalists and other holistic practitioners know that if a client comes in with many different health issues—and they're not sleeping well—helping the client sleep better will often resolve or mitigate many of the other concerns. Some people skimp on sleep because they don't prioritize it: the "I'll sleep when I'm dead" mentality. Others—likely most of you reading this book—want to get better sleep but are experiencing sleep problems. The good news is that herbs and a holistic approach will likely help us all sleep more soundly and have better vitality going forward.

The Importance of Sleep

Sleep is the ultimate panacea. During a good night's sleep, your body has the chance to relax muscles, repair damage, detoxify, fortify your immune system, balance out hormones and neurotransmitters, and restore itself. Getting adequate good-quality sleep is free, enjoyable, and one of the best things you can do to support your health. If you're coming down with a cold, dealing with a stressful period in your life, or trying to diet and lose weight, your day will go *much* more smoothly if you slept well the night before. Unfortunately, the reverse is also true.

LACK OF SLEEP = POOR HEALTH

We deteriorate with chronic sleep deprivation: Heart health, blood sugar metabolism, libido and reproductive health, psychological health, skin appearance, and our ability to maintain healthy habits all go to pieces. Just one or two nights of sleep deprivation diminishes our cognition, mood, and immune function. Sleeping less than 7 hours a night *triples* our risk of viral infection. On the other hand, if we get extra rest when we're sick, we'll recuperate more quickly.

Studies show that cutting down sleep to just 5 hours per night—instead of getting what is considered a well-rested 8 hours—can drive you to eat an additional 550 calories at night, makes it harder to stick to a healthy diet and make good self-care decisions, and can lead you to gain a whopping 2 pounds in just 5 days. Worse, British researchers found that workers who slept only 5 or fewer hours per night had double the risk of death from all causes versus those who averaged 7 or more hours. That "I'll sleep when I'm dead" mentality takes on new meaning! Most of us would rather get our beauty sleep and live longer, more vital lives.

In contrast to these dismal scenarios, getting adequate sleep improves almost every aspect of health. Aim for 7 to 9 hours of sleep per night for adults. You'll begin to reap the rewards almost immediately.

Having a hard time getting to sleep and staying there? Read on! In this book, we'll assess and address root causes of sleep disturbances and cover good sleep hygiene tips, and I'll share my favorite sleep-support herbs, remedies, and recipes.

How Sleep Works

A complex interplay of nervous system and endocrine (hormonal) system activity regulates your sleep–wake cycles, keeping you in balance day and night. Let's start with the key hormones: melatonin and cortisol.

THE SLEEP–WAKE CYCLE OF MELATONIN AND CORTISOL

Hormones are chemical messengers of the endocrine system that are excreted by endocrine glands and travel through your blood to interact with receptor sites throughout the body, before ultimately being converted into something new or broken down and excreted by the liver.

Melatonin. As you've likely heard, the hormone melatonin conducts the orchestra of sleep in our sleep–wake cycles. Melatonin is produced in the pineal gland in the brain in response to the darkening day. As the sun sets, your brain recognizes that night is falling and begins to increase melatonin levels, which reach

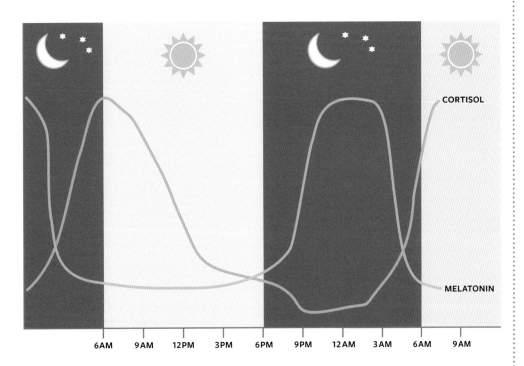

The hormones melatonin and cortisol regulate your sleep–wake cycles.

their highest levels around 1 to 3 a.m. Melatonin encourages various activities associated with rest, repair, and sedation, as well as immune function, downregulating inflammation, and more.

Cortisol. On the "wake" side of things is cortisol, a hormone produced in your adrenal glands. You've probably heard bad things about cortisol because it's a stress hormone associated with our nervous system's fight-or-flight response. But the key is balance. Cortisol is crucial for healthy body functioning and serves many essential purposes in the body.

In your daily cycles, cortisol should be at its lowest in the middle of the night, when your melatonin is the highest. As melatonin begins to wane in the early-morning hours, cortisol begins to rise. Cortisol should be the highest in the morning—that helps you get out of bed in the morning feeling energized—then it should gradually wane throughout the day and into night. When you experience disrupted sleep, it's possible that your melatonin and cortisol levels are out of balance.

Cortisol not only regulates our wake cycles, it's also essential for survival and kicks in when the body thinks that safety is being jeopardized. Cortisol is produced by the sympathetic nervous system as a stress response when you're in a fight-or-flight situation; it gives you the sustained energy to fight or flee. If your blood sugar dips too low between meals, a surge of cortisol tells your body to pull sugar from storage and put it into the bloodstream to tide you over and fuel your body. During sleep apnea, cortisol wakes you so you can get adequate oxygen.

Later in this book, as we discuss underlying triggers of insomnia, the concept of nighttime cortisol surges will be addressed. For now, just remember that we rely on the right amounts of cortisol at the right times of day for wakefulness, energy, and survival.

DARKNESS AND LIGHT

The *number one* factor regulating our healthy balance and timing of melatonin and cortisol for our sleep–wake cycle is *light*. We have evolved to respond to daylight (and firelight). When the level of light falling on our eyes and skin increases or decreases, that change tells our body which of our sleep–wake hormones to emphasize.

Our *culture* has evolved to bring artificial light into our daily lives through lamps, headlights, and TV, computer, and phone screens—and to spend dramatically less time outdoors during the day—but our *bodies* have *not* evolved to adapt to this influx of blue and superbright light. Studies show that when people spend time outdoors camping with no light except the sun and firelight, their sleep–wake cycles rapidly regain equilibrium. Even "night owls" go to bed earlier, wake earlier, and feel better rested. However, eschewing all screens and artificial light isn't practical for the lifestyles of most of us.

Tips to Support Sleep–Wake Cycles with Light

Our indoor lifestyles and exposure to artificial light and screens throw off our sleep–wake cycles and make it harder to unwind and sleep at night. If ditching artificial light and screens completely isn't practical, the following tips help to minimize their effects.

- **Turn off TV, phone, and computer screens at least 1 hour (ideally several hours) before bedtime.** For all ages, the light of devices as well as their content can be too stimulating and can derail sleep-supportive melatonin–cortisol balance. If you read at night, go for a regular book or use an e-reader that is not backlit, illuminating it from above with a small book light.

- **Dim the lights in your home and on your screens in the evening.** In our family, we love our twinkle lights. If you can, limit the nighttime use of LED bulbs, which emit blue light, and schedule your device screens to go into "night mode" at sunset, wear blue-light-blocking glasses, or install an app like f.lux.

- **Sleep in darkness to facilitate better melatonin and sleep.** Shut off all lights in the bedroom, install blackout curtains if needed, and consider wearing an eye mask, too.

- **Expose yourself to morning and midday sunlight.** Spend at least 10 minutes standing or exercising outside during the first half of the day. Don't stare directly at the sun, of course, but let your eyes see and skin feel daylight without sunglasses or windows for at least a portion of the day. Morning light helps set the schedule for your day's sleep–wake orchestra.

- **Choose "natural-feeling" lights.** Full-spectrum lights can provide circadian rhythm support by mimicking the sun's natural light; some lights will even slowly increase in intensity, to simulate the sunrise and wake you up in the morning.

- **Supplement with melatonin before bedtime.** This may also support your sleep cycle, though not as well as manipulating your relationship with light. See a deeper discussion on melatonin supplements on page 102.

Sleep by the Numbers

Survey reports show that, among adults:

- At least one-third don't get enough sleep.

- Two-thirds of women report frequent sleep problems.

- Women are two times more likely to experience sleep issues than men are.

- Certain ethnic groups, including Black women, are more significantly affected.

- People who are pregnant, postpartum, in later stages of perimenopause, and post-menopausal, as well as working moms, more often report new or worsening sleep problems.

- Surgical menopause (without hormone replacement) is associated with more than double the risk of sleep disruption versus natural menopause, as well as more intense symptoms.

- Eighty percent of women who reported sleeping poorly said they were also stressed, anxious, or worried, and 55 percent reported being sad, unhappy, or depressed. Daytime sleepiness is three times more prevalent, with many relying on caffeine to function, forgoing activities that promote health and joy.

- Americans who sleep less than 7 hours per night on weekdays are three times more likely to experience moderate to severe depression compared to those who sleep 7 to 9 hours.

- Other common disruptors of sleep include trauma and PTSD, working multiple jobs, being a single parent, caretaking, and sharing a bed with partners, children, or pets whose noise or movements disrupt sleep.

- Teens, who biologically need more sleep than adults, often shorten their sleep due to school, homework, social and extracurricular demands, and early-morning schedules. Teens average 2 hours less sleep per night than ideal for their age.

- Cognitive decline and sleep disruption are interlinked in many ways. Approximately 60 to 70 percent of people with cognitive impairment or dementia have sleep disturbances, and sleep difficulties tend to worsen cognition and increase cognitive disease prognosis. Common sleep medications also tend to worsen cognitive symptoms and the risk of dementia.

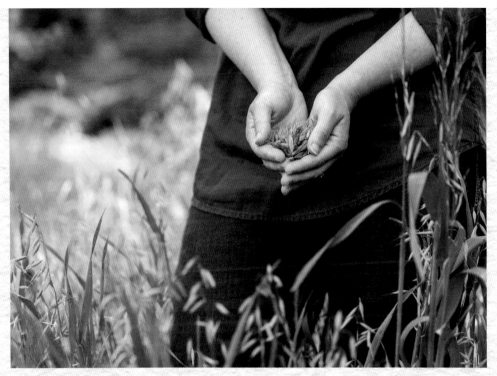

Milky oats nourish the nerves for long-term support of sleep, energy, and a healthy stress response.

- Thirty-four to 45 percent of adults in varying age groups reported unintentionally falling asleep during the day at least once in the past month—the highest numbers were for teens, young adults, seniors, and communities of color. Two to 7 percent reported having fallen asleep at the wheel in the past month—25- to 45-year-olds, men, and communities of color were most affected.

This is all to say that if you're experiencing stress, anxiety, and sleep difficulties, you're not alone. This book will guide you in how to sleuth out your own underlying triggers and find the herbs and lifestyle changes most likely to help you get a better night's sleep.

Core Habits for Better Sleep

It can be hard to get out of an insomnia rut. In addition to regulating sleep–wake cycles by adjusting your light exposure (discussed on page 5), here are some of the core general strategies to support your relaxation and sleep cycle.

DE-STRESS

Stress is a major factor in most cases of insomnia. Calming or sedative herbs at night and/or stress-relieving herbs during the day can help, but also try to reduce the stressors directly. Maybe you need to back out of stressful situations (for example, a bad job or relationship, having said yes when you should have said no) or schedule more rest-and-relaxation time for yourself. Consider regular meditation, yoga, daytime exercise, or an evening wind-down ritual of reading and sipping tea. Add relaxing herbs to the kids' nighttime baths. We'll talk more about stress and relaxation support and herbs later in this book.

DEVELOP A SLEEP RITUAL

Parents of young children know that consistency and ritual make all the difference. After you've unplugged (see page 5), get ready for bed and get comfy! Enjoy a small cup of relaxing tea or warm milk with honey (but not so much that you'll have to pee at midnight or go on a blood sugar roller coaster). Good pre-bed activities include reading a book (but *not* a page-turning suspense novel), journaling (a good time for that gratitude journal!), making love, listening to calming music, cuddling up with loved ones, meditating, inhaling relaxing essential oils or incense, and taking a bath.

Turn your bedroom into a sanctuary. Make it a soothing place to relax and sleep—but not much else. Having a cooler bedroom but warm feet and blankets often supports sleep. Earplugs help if it's noisy. I love my eye mask!

AVOID OR MODERATE STIMULANTS

Stimulants of various sorts can make you restless and more apt to wake up. Examples of stimulants and stimulating experiences include the following.

Caffeine. Coffee, chocolate, yerba maté, soda, and green and black tea are obvious late-night no-nos, but you may be surprised by the effect that even morning caffeine has. Cut down slowly (to avoid withdrawal headaches)—or go cold turkey and deal with a few days of misery (hydration helps!)—to see if sleep improves. You may be okay with a morning cuppa, but opt for naturally

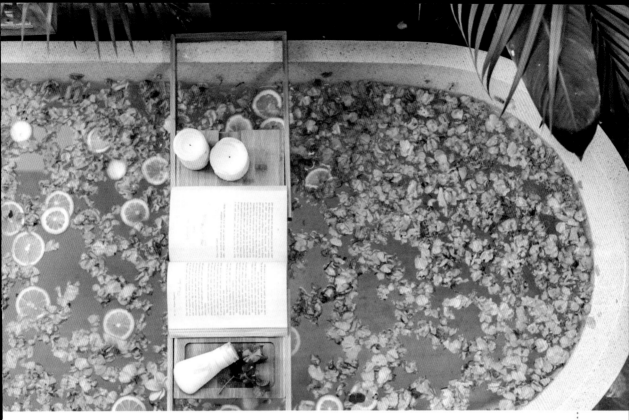

Creating a relaxing bedtime ritual—whether simple or elaborate—can help you unwind and shift toward better sleep cycles.

caffeine-free options after noon, such as tulsi, golden milk, herbal chai, lemon balm tea with fresh lemon juice, and seltzer. (See Chapter 6 for recipe ideas.)

Medications, herbs, and supplements. Even if they don't contain caffeine, many remedies can cause restlessness, especially if you take them later in the day. This includes B vitamins and multivitamins, stimulant adaptogens, testosterone and most testosterone-supporting herbs, ADHD meds, some blood pressure medications, antidepressants, dementia medications, antihistamines, asthma medications, glucosamine and chondroitin, and statins. Try switching herbs and supplements around or avoid late doses. Always talk with your doctor first if you suspect medications are the cause of your wakefulness to see if it's safe and appropriate to try a different medication or change your dose time. Sensitive people may find that adaptogenic herbs, adaptogen-like mushrooms (like chaga and cordyceps, possibly reishi), and "detoxifying" herbs disrupt sleep. (For more on adaptogens, see Chapter 2.)

ALTER YOUR LIFESTYLE

These foundational changes can lead to big improvements in sleep quality!

Lay off the booze. Alcohol may initially sedate but ultimately makes you restless, disrupts blood sugar, aggravates sleep apnea, and prevents restful deep sleep. As we age or transition through menopause, we become even more sensitive to alcohol's sleep-disrupting activities. Even one or two drinks might be too many.

Avoid late-night eating. Late or heavy dinners and snack binges wreak havoc on a good night's sleep; blood sugar roller coasters, active digestion, and liver involvement can affect you for several hours after you eat. Try to stop eating at least 4 hours before bedtime and particularly avoid big, heavy dishes and sugar- or fat-laden food. Many people sleep best fasting for 12 to 16 hours between dinner and breakfast—with an emphasis on earlier dinner rather than later breakfast.

Exercise during the day. Physical activity is *phenomenal* for addressing insomnia and stress. But not right before bedtime—aim for morning or midday activity instead. That said, late-day exercise is better than none.

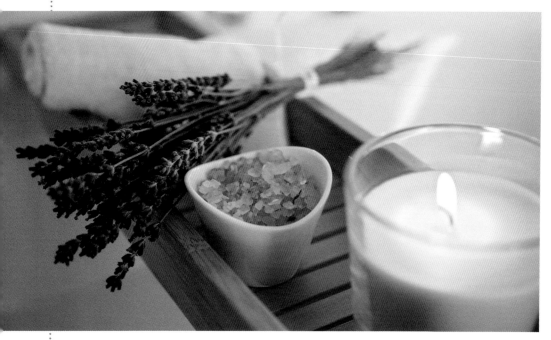

Turning down artificial lights at night and inhaling relaxing aromas like lavender help tell your body it's time for bed.

Understanding and Supporting Quality Sleep

I *Still* Can't Sleep! What's Going On?

Perhaps you've made all the aforementioned core sleep hygiene changes, and you still aren't sleeping well. It can be incredibly frustrating to be in a vicious cycle of insomnia that doesn't respond to the usual tricks, sleep herbs, or melatonin. It's always important to address the *root cause* of insomnia, otherwise herbs may not work or may work briefly and then stop working.

Many factors may underlie your inability to get quality sleep—particularly if you wake in the middle of the night in alarm mode, unable to fall back to sleep, but also if you have difficulties falling asleep. Common culprits include sleep apnea, blood sugar dysregulation, menopausal hormone shifts, and ongoing stress or trauma. Other factors may also underlie sleep issues. It's *always* a good idea to talk to your doctor to see if a sleep study and ruling out other more serious conditions are appropriate.

SLEEP APNEA

The likelihood of developing sleep apnea, and its severity and that of related conditions, increases with age, weight gain, menopause, alcohol, sedatives, mouth breathing, a narrow palate, sleeping on your back, and food or environmental allergens. During sleep apnea, the structure of the airway relaxes and shifts, inhibiting or cutting off oxygen. The body *needs* oxygen, so it kicks into survival mode, surging cortisol to wake you up so you can breathe. You may not realize it's happening.

Signs of sleep apnea. People with sleep apnea often snore and are heavier set, but not always. Other signs that suggest sleep apnea include waking with a dry mouth, sore throat, or headache, and waking feeling unrefreshed. You may feel sluggish, sleepy, and doze off during the day. The bodily stress of sleep apnea and lack of oxygen at night ultimately increases your risk of cardiovascular disease, hypertension, blood sugar instability, weight gain, increased appetite for junk food, cognitive decline, depression, car accidents, and a shorter life span. Don't ignore it! Ask your doctor for a sleep study, which is the best way to diagnose apnea. Though less reliable, at-home kits to test oxygen levels throughout the night or an app that listens to you breathe or tracks your body's movements may suggest the presence of the disorder.

Choosing the right treatment. Sedating herbs and drugs are likely to make the problem *worse* by further relaxing the airway muscles and making it harder for your body to wake to get

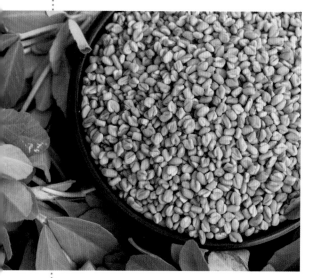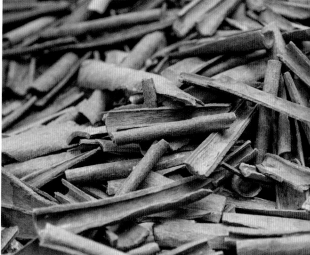

Fenugreek seeds (left) modulate glucose and insulin in a wide range of blood sugar situations. Cinnamon (right) specifically enhances sensitivity of cells to insulin, which is helpful in insulin resistance and some early stages of pre-diabetes and type 2 diabetes.

life-supporting oxygen. Gentle nervine and adaptogenic herbs—which we'll cover in this book—are less likely to worsen apnea, but they won't address it. If your case is mild, it *may* respond to sleeping on your side, losing weight, propping the head of your bed up a few inches, and addressing any of your personal triggers from the above list. But the best therapy for sleep apnea is a CPAP machine or similar device. Once you get used to the device, the changes in your body will be remarkable—increased vitality, better mood, better cognition, better sleep, and so much more.

BLOOD SUGAR DYSREGULATION

Even if you don't have diabetes or pre-diabetes, odds are you have some level of blood sugar dysregulation. A 2022 study reviewing 2018 data determined that 93 percent of US adults had less-than-optimal cardiometabolic (combined cardiovascular and blood sugar) health—that's huge! Blood sugar levels and increased adipose (fat) tissue had particularly worsened from the prior years' data, and these numbers have probably gotten even worse in more recent years. Dysregulated blood sugar is a big topic, but let's focus here on how it affects sleep.

Understanding and Supporting Quality Sleep

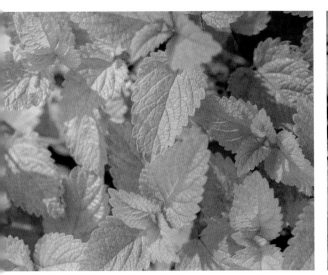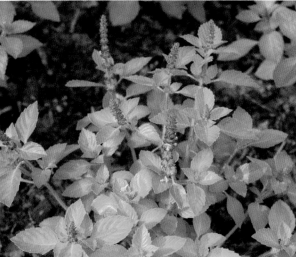

Lemon balm (left) and holy basil (right) offer calming yet uplifting benefits alongside mild glucose reduction. They're particularly helpful during stress-induced glucose roller coasters and cravings.

When you eat foods that contain starch and sugar, your blood sugar (glucose) naturally increases, and insulin releases from beta cells to help it get into your cells and muscles to fuel the body's energy production. Eventually, glucose and insulin dip back down until the next meal. Diabetes is diagnosed when you regularly test over 100 mg/dL (milligrams per deciliter) for fasting glucose or 200 mg/dL on a random glucose test. But *optimal* fasting glucose is between 75 and 85 mg/dL, and you feel best if glucose doesn't spike more than 30 mg/dL from its starting point after you eat. Most people fall outside of these ranges and experience repercussions, including sleep disruption.

The blood sugar roller coaster. Dysregulated blood sugar often occurs due to consuming too much sugar and quick-release starches. Glucose levels leap to high levels with big spikes, and cells become resistant to insulin because they're overwhelmed with the fuel overload. Excess glucose gets shoved into storage in fat cells, which accumulate throughout the body—particularly in the abdomen. Glucose is also turned into triglycerides and LDL cholesterol, accumulates as fat in the liver, and is excreted in the urine. The gentle rolling hills of healthy glucose and insulin levels turn into a frightening roller coaster with big spikes followed by hypoglycemic crashes, that, ironically, make us crave *more* sugar and simple carbs.

How blood sugar dysregulation can disrupt sleep. When blood sugar crashes after a spike, cortisol kicks in to tell your body to pull sugar from storage and put it into the bloodstream. It also drives your hunger to eat more sugar and carbs. Midnight blood sugar crashes after nighttime sweets and snacks—followed by a surge of energizing cortisol—are a cause of waking in the middle of the night. You might remember that this survival stress hormone also regulates the wake part of our sleep–wake cycles. Cortisol also surges when you're stressed or experiencing sleep apnea, and—as we'll cover shortly—during hot flashes.

Strategies and herbs that help. The best way to address blood sugar dysregulation is to "flatten your glucose curve" throughout the day by eating high-fiber whole carbs in moderation alongside veggies, protein, and healthy fats, and being particularly mindful about nighttime intake of sugar, simple carbs, and excessive food. For helpful "glucose flattening" tips, see Jessie Inchauspé's book *Glucose Revolution* and her Instagram page (see Resources, page 178). You can monitor your progress with at-home morning fasting finger-prick tests or a continuous glucose monitor; you'll also notice improvements in your energy and vitality when your blood sugar is in balance.

Herbs that support glucose balance include cinnamon, fenugreek, magnolia, hops, lemon balm, and holy basil (see Resources, page 178, to learn more). *Always* check with your doctor *before* adding herbs or making big diet changes, *especially* if you have diabetes and/or take insulin or glucose-regulating medications, to ensure safety. Consider also working alongside a nutritionist, herbalist, and/or naturopathic doctor for holistic support.

MENOPAUSE AND AGING

This is a topic near and dear to my heart as a postmenopausal woman who works with many clients who are challenged by menopausal changes. During menopause your natural production of estrogen, progesterone, and melatonin wanes, which makes you more sensitive to the effects of stress hormones. The reduction of estrogen also makes you more susceptible to blood sugar dysregulation, weight gain, reduced bladder tone, and sleep apnea. That's because estrogen and progesterone have a protective influence on mood, glucose regulation, and tone. In surgical menopause, the hormone shifts and sleep disruption tend to be even more severe.

Hot flashes. These also kick in as estrogen wobbles and drops off in late

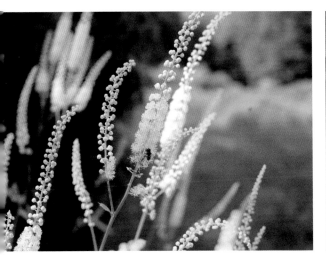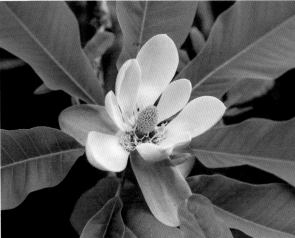

Herbs like black cohosh (left) and magnolia (right) may support sleep by balancing various hormones that affect our sleep quality, such as estrogen and cortisol.

perimenopause and postmenopause. Hot flashes can be triggered by temperature changes, stress, and stress hormones. During a hot flash, you also experience a brief surge of cortisol and stress hormones that may manifest as agitation, anxiety, and heart palpitations alongside a few minutes of hot sweaty mess . . . and this can wake you up if you're sleeping. Peri- and postmenopausal people who have higher levels of inflammation, glucose dysregulation, body weight, prior reproductive health issues (like endometriosis), sleep apnea, stress, and trauma are more likely to experience hot flashes.

The sleep disruption of menopause is particularly acute *during* the hot flash, but the effects reach beyond the hot flash itself. Low estrogen increases sensitivity to stress hormones, anxiety, and glucose dysregulation, as well as reduced melatonin production, and causes greater susceptibility to insomnia triggers—such as stimulants, caffeine, screen time, alcohol, and nighttime snacking—than you had during your prime reproductive years.

Interestingly, in people born with ovaries, higher testosterone levels are often correlated with insulin resistance and polycystic ovarian syndrome, but in people born with testes, insulin resistance develops when testosterone drops. So, we may see similar patterns in andropause and PCOS, too.

Strategies and herbs that help. Thankfully, it's possible to restore balance to these challenging situations. Some of the most helpful approaches include:

* Supporting a healthier stress and relaxation response (see Chapters 3 and 4).

* Eating a healthy whole foods plant-based or Mediterranean-style diet, which will help reduce inflammation and flatten glucose curves.

* Taking menopausal hormone-supportive herbs, such as shatavari, black cohosh, fenugreek, white peony root, magnolia, and hops. I love formulas that combine some of these reproductive herbs with adaptogens and nervines by day and more relaxing herbs at night. I tend to recommend hops (featured on page 99) only at night because it's so sedating. While magnolia (page 40) and peony root are nice day *and* night, they have additional sleep-support benefits.

In surgical menopause, relaxing herbs as well as black cohosh (which is safe for people at risk for estrogen-sensitive cancers) and shatavari may help. In some cases, estrogen medication may be the best option for sleep and hot flashes, with side benefits for cognition and bone strength. However, other variables—including increasing the risk of estrogen-dependent cancer or blood clots, and masculine gender affirmation—may make estrogen less appropriate. Talk with your doctor to assess risks and benefits to determine what's right for you. (Also see Recommended Reading, page 177, for books covering reproductive hormone balance in depth.)

STRESS, WORRY, AND TRAUMA

We mentioned stress on pages 4 and 8, and we'll come back to it again in Chapter 2. But it bears repeating here: Stress, worry, and trauma can *profoundly* disrupt sleep and interplay with other triggers and root causes, including blood sugar levels and hot flashes. I've witnessed countless examples of sleep challenges during times of stress, trauma, grief, or worry. Once again, cortisol and our stress hormones interfere, and then the lack of sleep makes us more susceptible to daytime stress and mood instability in a vicious cycle.

Strategies and herbs that help. Alongside the herbs and approaches we'll cover in Chapters 3 and 4 as well as the recipes in Chapter 6, I urge you to give yourself extra TLC and honor your need for self-care, downtime, and healing. Devote time to activities that bring you joy and peace. Also consider seeking the support of a therapist. Many types of therapy exist. Some people find great value in learning to shift their habits and thinking processes with cognitive-behavioral therapy. Others prefer the opportunity to discuss their history and concerns through traditional talk therapy. For trauma, finding a high-quality trauma-informed therapist can be invaluable. You may find talk therapy, energizing herbs, sedatives, and meditation triggering in early and acute trauma stages and may prefer art, music, movement, and nervine herbs. For more tips, check out Elizabeth Guthrie's *The Trauma Informed Herbalist* book and podcast, as well as the upcoming chapters of this book.

PAIN

Chronic pain afflicts 100 million people in the United States—nearly four times the number of people affected by diabetes, and more than diabetes, heart disease, and cancer combined. Pain and sleep difficulties fuel each other. Sleep problems occur in 67 to 88 percent of people suffering with chronic pain disorders. Pain management and resolution approaches will vary based on the person and root cause of pain. Your support team might include a conventional doctor, holistic practitioner, bodywork, and/or physical therapy. Generally supportive lifestyle changes to reduce inflammation include regular exercise and stretching (that doesn't aggravate your injury);

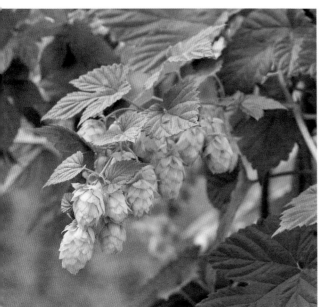 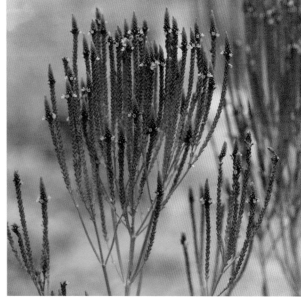

Hops (left) and blue vervain (right) are two herbs that help relieve pain in different ways while also relaxing the mind to support sleep.

an anti-inflammatory and glucose-supportive diet rich in plant foods, lean protein, magnesium, and omega-3s; and mind–body balance, which I'll discuss in more depth in Chapter 3.

Strategies and herbs that help. Many herbs support sleep, decrease stress, and help ease inflammation, pain, and muscle tension. Of these, ashwagandha, holy basil, blue vervain, wood betony, magnolia, and tart cherry are generally helpful day or night. Save the more sedating pain-relieving herbs—such as California poppy, hops, valerian, and Jamaican dogwood—for bedtime. Whether cannabis is suitable for day or night depends on the variety; each strain has a different amount and type of terpenes and cannabinoids.

Consider blending these relaxing pain-support herbs with more straightforward anti-inflammatory and pain-relief herbs, including turmeric, ginger, cinnamon, boswellia, Solomon's seal, mullein root, horsetail, meadowsweet, willow and poplar species, peony root, homeopathic or topical arnica, and low-dose corydalis. You'll want to learn more about each herb because they have affinities for different types of pain. (For deeper discussions on natural and herbal pain management, refer to the Recommended Reading list on page 177.)

NIGHTTIME URINATION

As we age, we have a greater risk of urination problems that disrupt a full night's sleep—no matter our gender. Needing to get up to pee once, or even twice, as we age is normal. However, it can also be frustrating. The reasons for nocturnal urination vary and can include overhydration in the evening, benign prostatic hyperplasia, reduction of bladder tone, and other challenges. Changes

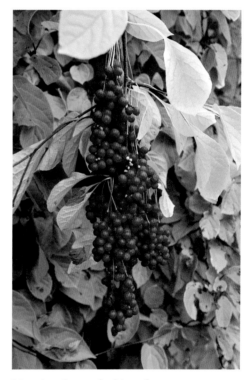

Morning doses of schizandra may support energy, healthy stress response, and balanced sleep while also reducing leaky fluids in the body.

Understanding and Supporting Quality Sleep

to the anatomy while giving birth and during menopause can affect urinary and bladder tone, though younger people may also experience problems. Nighttime cortisol surges—from hot flashes, stress, blood sugar crashes, or sleep apnea—may also increase the need to pee, because our body thinks it's time to wake up.

Strategies and herbs that help. Addressing the underlying root cause is important, as well as focusing on hydrating during the day and limiting liquids at night. Physical therapy can be quickly and dramatically helpful. Certain herbs and supplements may also support bladder and prostate tone, including melatonin or theanine (both discussed on pages 102 and 103 as sleep-supportive supplements), pumpkin seeds, pumpkin seed oil, schizandra (during the day), nettle root (during the day), mullein root, and possibly herbs that are soothing to the urinary tract, such as marshmallow root and corn silk. As always, research these options further and talk with your healthcare provider before integrating them into your routine. In some situations, surgery may be necessary, and prostate issues should be monitored by your doctor.

RESTLESS LEGS SYNDROME (RLS)

This neurological sleep disorder can be maddening, not only for the person experiencing it but also for their bedpartner(s). Consider getting everything checked by your doctor first to rule out underlying causes, such as iron deficiency and kidney, spinal cord, or neurological problems. For most people RLS is simply an annoyance.

Strategies and herbs that help. Nerve-calming herbs at night may help, such as passionflower, skullcap, blue vervain, and California poppy. Also try supporting hydration and electrolytes, including sodium, potassium, calcium,

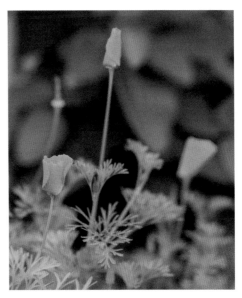

California poppy calms the mind and the nerves to promote slumber.

When to See a Doctor or Holistic Practitioner

If you're having trouble sleeping, it's *always* a good idea to mention it to your doctor so that you can pinpoint issues together and rule out important underlying causes that may require medical attention. This is especially true if insomnia has persisted for several weeks or is interfering with your daytime functioning or mental health. A sleep study may be helpful. Holistic practitioners such as herbalists and naturopathic doctors can also be helpful additions to your team—they will be able to guide you in your herbal and natural remedy options and help you avoid herb–drug interactions. Herbalists typically have a more nuanced understanding of plant medicine and are better able to customize your herbal care and teach you how to make your own remedies; however, they cannot diagnose, prescribe, or make recommendations on your pharmaceuticals. If your sleep and health issues are complicated or your sleep is unresponsive to herbal remedies at home, consider seeking professional support. Keep your doctor and pharmacist in the loop on the natural approaches you're taking. For additional tips for people taking medications, see page 166. For herb safety in children, pregnancy, and lactation, see page 169.

and magnesium throughout the day, especially if your RLS is triggered by physical activity. Some people find simply sipping tomato juice or calcium-rich milk, or eating a banana, eases symptoms. Homeopathic remedies for restless legs may also help.

OTHER CONDITIONS

These are *some* of the most common underlying causes of sleep issues that may also respond well to herbs, but it's not an exhaustive list. Complex conditions include fibromyalgia, active Epstein-Barr virus, chronic fatigue syndrome, long COVID, and chronic/post-acute Lyme. Neurological and mental health conditions, thyroid problems (particularly hyperthyroid), anemia, and respiratory and cardiovascular disease may also be present. Many of the herbs and approaches in this book may be supportive but won't fully address the underlying issues. Seek the assistance of a doctor for diagnosis and medical care, if needed, and a holistic practitioner to guide your natural medicine journey with these challenging and multifaceted conditions.

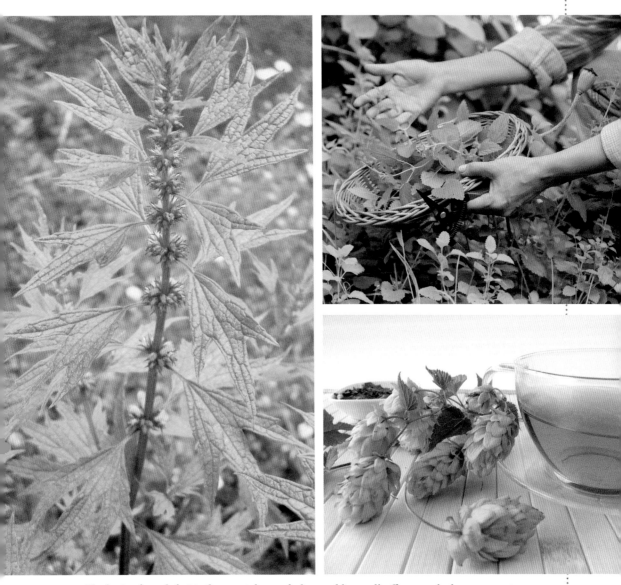

Clockwise from left: Motherwort, lemon balm, and hops all offer superb sleep support and calming properties—each with different attributes that can make one or another more appropriate for different people or different times of day.

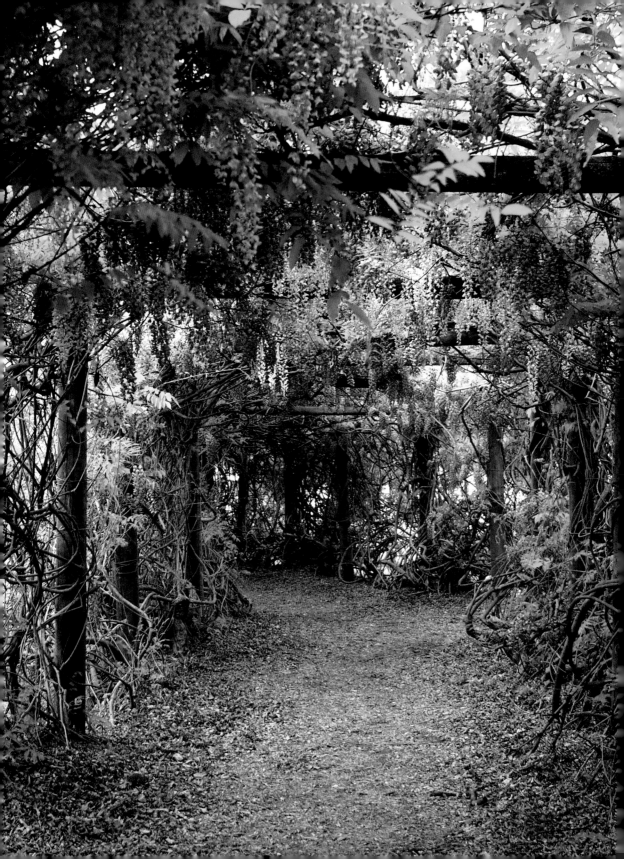

CHAPTER 2

Managing Stress and Daytime Energy

If you feel like stress interferes with your quality of life and sleep, you're not alone. More than 75 percent of Americans are regularly stressed. Common stressors include work, money, relationships and family, grief, trauma, loneliness, health, sleep deprivation, poor nutrition, and media overload. These and other stressors can put your nervous system's responses into overdrive, which sets off a chain of bad reactions throughout your body. The good news? Healthy habits and herbs can help flip the switch in your favor.

The Effects of Stress

The term *stress* can mean many things. Most often, it refers to the sympathetic nervous system's fight-or-flight response. An interconnected surge of neurotransmitters (nervous system) and stress hormones (endocrine system) triggers widespread effects throughout your body to help you meet the demands of the perceived threat, either by fighting or by fleeing, which has many downstream effects, including disrupted sleep.

THE GOOD SIDE

The foremost result of stress is a burst of energy, which was crucial in helping our ancestors fight or flee from imminent threats like large wild beasts. Today we may even enjoy and rely on those quick bursts of stress-induced energy. Other positive effects of short-term stress include the following.

* Increased brain activity

* Expanded airways

* Increased heart strength

* Increased blood flow to the organs involved in fighting and fleeing

THE BAD SIDE

Your body isn't meant to sustain the stress response over the long term, and doing so causes wear and tear on many body systems. Some of the negative effects of long-term stress include the following.

* Cognition and memory issues

* Insomnia

* Fatigue and/or feeling "wired"

* Depression and/or anxiety

* Systemic inflammation

* Decreased blood flow to the periphery and the rest-and-repair organs

* Poor metabolism, including elevated cortisol and blood sugar, which can lead to diabetes and abdominal weight gain

* Slow digestion, indigestion, gas, pain, bloating, irritable bowel syndrome, and/or constipation

* Increased blood viscosity and clotting, pressure on the cardiovascular system including endothelial inflammation, high blood pressure, high cholesterol levels, and increased risk of stroke

* Decreased libido and impaired reproductive health and function

* Decreased detoxification

* Decreased immune function

* Slower, less effective wound healing and reduced connective tissue integrity

Managing Stress and Daytime Energy

So, you can see how just one little thing—stress—can affect your entire well-being and factor into a range of diseases. Both short- and long-term stress affect sleep quality. In my clinical practice, chronic stress is a *major* player in most of my clients' health concerns and general state of vitality. Simply addressing stress levels and helping the body balance stress hormones can correct or reduce the severity of conditions that may not otherwise seem related.

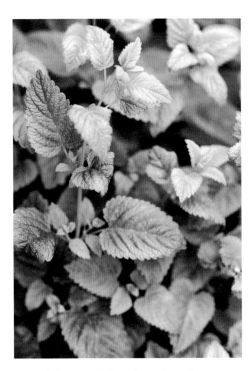

One of the most beloved nervines, lemon balm eases stress by nourishing and calming the nervous system.

COMPOUNDS THAT DRIVE THE STRESS RESPONSE

Because stress played an integral role in humans' early survival, the compounds that elicit the stress response are incredibly potent. Most of our stress chemicals—the key adrenal hormones—are produced by the adrenal gland as well as the nervous system. Adrenaline (also known as epinephrine) functions as both a neurotransmitter and a hormone. Why is this important? Neurotransmitters travel through your nervous system quickly, jumping from synapse to synapse, which triggers a lightning-fast response. Enzymes break neurotransmitters down very quickly, too, which means the effects are short-lived.

In contrast, hormones travel through your blood, acting on cell receptor sites. Hormones move more slowly than neurotransmitters and take longer to be broken down and eliminated (via liver detoxification). Eventually, the stress hormone cortisol gets in on the action, releasing sugar from storage into your bloodstream to fuel the perceived stress demands and shifting your levels of energy and fatigue, wakefulness and sleepiness, and metabolism. Excessive or dysregulated stress chemicals easily disrupt sleep–wake cycles and challenge our sleep quality.

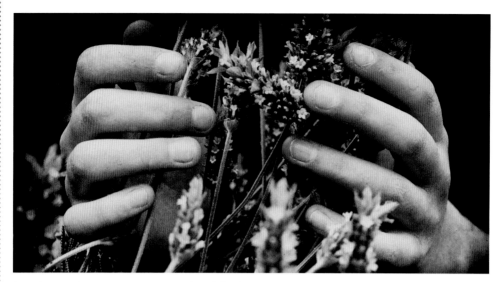

Simply spending time in nature and with herbs can improve our stress response—especially when it's with a relaxing herb like lavender.

ADDRESSING CHRONIC STRESS

These stress-related compounds are an essential part of health, but chronic stress throws them out of whack and pulls your body out of balance quickly. If you really were responding to a primal source of stress like a saber-toothed tiger, the physical acts of fighting or fleeing would help clear these stress hormones from your system more quickly. However, modern sources of stress don't generally give you a physical outlet. This is one reason why chronic stress causes so much damage across your body systems—and it explains why regular exercise does a nice job of decreasing the effects of stress and why we tend to sleep better when we exercise earlier in the day.

Addressing your personal stress culprits is the main goal. You can do a number of things in your routine—from quitting a terrible job and saying no more often to taking up a regular meditation practice and exercising regularly—to reduce your stress levels. Addressing these modern culprits has the most meaningful and long-term impact on stress and well-being. But to support yourself in the journey, you can turn to herbs that help the body adapt to stress, and you can also encourage your body to return to the parasympathetic nervous system's rest-and-repair state. Enter the wonderful world of adaptogens.

Managing Stress and Daytime Energy

Supporting the Stress Response with Adaptogens

Adaptogens help your body adapt to stress and usually have an energizing effect. Soviet researcher Nikolai Vasilyevich Lazarev coined the term in the mid-1940s, and the concept was researched heavily in the region during that time. The plants we now call adaptogens have a long history of aiding longevity and vitality throughout antiquity and across the globe. Adaptogens are defined by their actions.

* They're relatively nontoxic and safe, supporting well-being.

* They have beneficial effects on a range of body systems, nourishing and balancing them. They affect not only stress and energy but often also fertility, libido, reproductive hormone balance, immune vitality, longevity, and mood.

* They often have a modulating effect. For example, depending on whether levels of a particular hormone are low or high, an adaptogen may increase or decrease the body's production of that hormone.

* They seem to work by affecting the stress response and the hypothalamic-pituitary-adrenal axis of the neuroendocrine system's production of stress-related neurotransmitters and hormones.

* Newer science suggests that adaptogens also improve mitochondrial function to enhance energy production on a cellular level, and many also enhance oxygen utilization.

To put it more simply, adaptogenic herbs help your body adapt so that you have a more balanced response to stress.

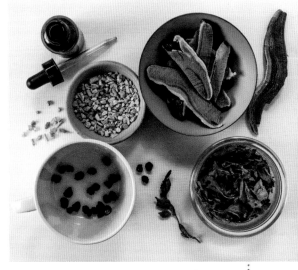

Popular, safe, sustainably available adaptogens to support a healthy stress response and sleep–wake cycles include (clockwise from top right) reishi mushroom, holy basil, schizandra berries, and ashwagandha. They can be helpful daytime allies.

When you take these herbs, you're less apt to jump into fight-or-flight mode yet still have better overall energy and ability to deal with the stress. Compared to the other herbs in this book, adaptogens are more stimulating in nature, but they're not overt stimulants like caffeine. Adaptogens are more balancing and restorative for the stress response and many other body systems as well.

We turn to adaptogens for a range of conditions whenever stress is a primary or underlying factor—which it often is! They are especially helpful when stress has left you feeling fatigued and sluggish (physically or mentally) and when daytime stress and dysregulated cortisol function make it hard to sleep at night. When supporting sleep, we often incorporate adaptogens *earlier* in the day, such as with breakfast, and focus on more calming herbs—the nervines, relaxants, and sedatives we'll discuss in the next two chapters—at night.

ADAPTOGENS FOR SLEEP SUPPORT

As a general rule, adaptogens tend to be somewhat stimulating. Even though they're more restorative than overt stimulants, their effects on sleep quality are varied. There is a continuum of adaptogens, from "more zippy" (like ginseng and rhodiola) to "more calming" (like ashwagandha and holy basil). Yet different people may also respond differently to each adaptogen.

For example, I find schizandra balancing and eleuthero agitating, yet some of my fellow herbalists experience the opposite. When my students discuss holy basil and ashwagandha, it's amazing how our experiences vary with the same plant—from "It helps me get up and go!" to "I feel too high or relaxed to work." It's always important to listen to your body to determine how *you* experience each plant and which plants resonate most for you.

When it comes to sleep support, as a general rule, opt for the more calming and balancing adaptogens rather than the zippier, stimulating ones. The more calming adaptogens help balance the stress responses in a broad spectrum of people and conditions. They simultaneously energize and calm. These herbs also have some very useful side benefits, and they are well

Managing Stress and Daytime Energy

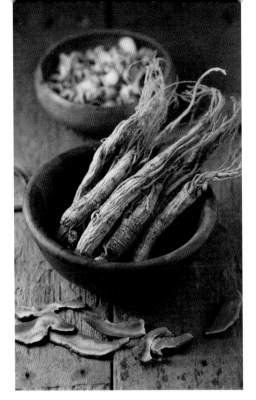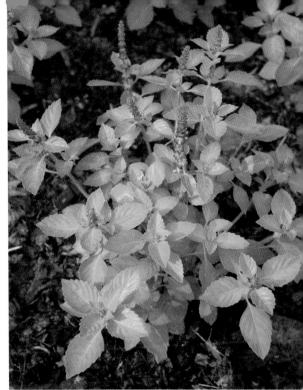

Although ginseng (left) is a classic adaptogenic herb, its stimulating qualities, sustainability issues, rampant adulteration, and high price has me turning more often to holy basil (right), which is often better for sleep and is easy to grow in the garden.

tolerated, which makes them extremely useful in formulas. I turn to them more often than any others when supporting my clients with sleep issues or anxiety.

Some of my favorite balancing adaptogens and adaptogen-like herbs and mushrooms that help us regulate healthy sleep–wake cycles include ashwagandha, holy basil, magnolia, reishi, schizandra, shatavari, and gotu kola. Each plant has its own nuances, considerations, and side benefits.

A note about timing: Consider incorporating adaptogens—especially the zippier ones like ashwagandha and schizandra—earlier in the day, such as with breakfast. By having a healthier stress response during the day, it will generally be easier to wind down at night.

Also be sure to see the tips for taking herbs in Chapter 6, page 118. For additional safety tips, including for children and for those who are taking medications, pregnant, or lactating, see Chapter 7.

Ashwagandha

Withania somnifera
Nightshade Family (Solanaceae)

 Appropriate during the daytime. Unlikely to impair function; may have moderately energizing activity.

 Well balanced, with effects that are generally helpful day or night. Unlikely to oversedate by day or overstimulate at night.

According to ancient wisdom in the system of Ayurveda in India, taking ashwagandha regularly for a year will give you the strength of a stallion for the next 10 years. Consider ashwagandha when the nervous-adrenal system needs to be nourished and restored. It supports deep energy, as well as sleep. Ashwagandha is one of my favorite herbs for myself and clients. You often see results within a few days, with further improvement over time.

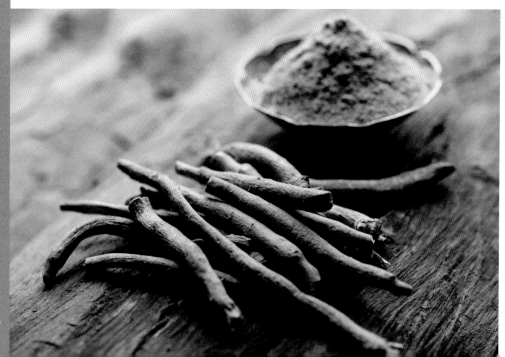

An Adaptogen for Sleep

In spite of ashwagandha's energizing effects, it's also a popular sleep aid. The species name *somnifera* means "sleep-inducing." The deeply restorative qualities of ashwagandha for the nervous system and sleep particularly shine in hot milk. Ashwagandha can also be helpful for people who are dealing with trauma and PTSD. But whether ashwagandha is more overtly calming or energizing—as well as the best form, dose, and time of day—is also *highly individual*. Some people find it overstimulating and that it aggravates insomnia and anxiety, while others feel deeply relaxed.

Multifaceted Restoration

This aromatic root supports not only deep energy, calm mind, and better sleep but also physical strength, perky and stable mood, cognitive prowess, increased muscle mass, nourished nerves, less pain and inflammation, reduced cancer risk, healthy immune and respiratory systems, upregulated thyroid function, increased libido, enhanced hormones and fertility, and more. It's often helpful for fatigue in autoimmune and chronic disease states, such as long COVID, fibromyalgia, and chronic Lyme. Ashwagandha benefits all genders yet has an affinity for testosterone support and sperm vitality.

Formulate It with Fat

Although ashwagandha works well in many different formats, Ayurvedic practitioners often stir the powder into hot milk (cow, coconut, or almond), ghee, or another warm, fatty substance, based on the belief that this would better send ashwagandha to the fat-lined nervous system. It's a great addition to "golden milk," which is traditionally made with turmeric, honey, hot milk, and a pinch of black pepper. I add a pinch each of cardamom and nutmeg and sometimes blend in egg and vanilla extract (eggnog!). Any fatty "milk" will do; if you avoid conventional dairy, try almond, full-fat oat milk, or coconut milk.

Ashwagandha tastes okay—earthy, nutty, raw-potato, woodsy—and you can add some honey or maple syrup and sweet spices to make it even tastier. Ashwagandha blends well in decocted teas, including chai, and with cocoa powder.

Safety and Considerations

Ashwagandha is safe for most people, with some cautions. If you have sensitivities to nightshade-family plants such as tomatoes, potatoes, eggplant, and peppers, be aware that ashwagandha is also in this plant family; however, it is less likely to trigger sensitivities. Because it may stimulate thyroid function, avoid it in hyperthyroid disease and seek guidance before combining it with thyroid-boosting medications like

ASHWAGANDHA

Synthroid, Cytomel, or thyroid glandulars—in these situations, there is a risk of dangerous overstimulation of the thyroid. This may manifest as agitation, anxiety, insomnia, palpitations, and feeling overheated, as well as thyroid hormone changes on labs—low or lowish TSH (thyroid-stimulating hormone), possibly higher free T3 and free T4 (both of which are specific types of thyroid hormones). Other herb–drug interactions are possible but rare. Don't use it during pregnancy without professional supervision. If you have iron overload, do not use ashwagandha—the root bioaccumulates iron from the soil; however, tinctures are typically safe because alcohol doesn't extract minerals.

Working with Ashwagandha

I prefer to work with dried ashwagandha roots, though some herbalists also work with the fresh root and, for different attributes, the aerial parts. In my experience, Indian-grown ashwagandha—most often available commercially—is more stimulating compared to ashwagandha purchased direct from US herb farms or grown in the backyard. Preference is highly individual. It can be grown in cooler climates and harvested in just one growing season.

Part used: roots

Tea or hot milk: ¼–1 teaspoon powdered or 1 tablespoon cut/sifted roots per cup, simmered 10+ minutes, one to three times daily

Tincture: 1–5 mL, one to three times daily, solo or in formula

Dried 1:5 in 50–60 percent alcohol

Powder/capsules: 1–6 g per day in capsules or mixed into hot milk, ghee, honey, or spice blends

Recipes: Ashwagandha Chai, page 132 • Adaptogen Chai "Mule" (variation), page 132 • Adaptogen "Coffee," page 134 • Adaptogen Frozen Iced "Coffee" (variation), page 134 • Ashwagandha Golden Milk, page 139 • Stress Relief Tincture Blend, page 148 • Mellow Me Glycerite, page 152

Growing and Harvesting Ashwagandha

Ashwagandha is a tender perennial (USDA Zones 8–11) that can be grown like an annual in cool climates. Grow it as you would tomatoes: Ashwagandha loves heat, sun, and well-drained soil (rich to sandy) without competition from nearby plants. Start seeds indoors (they are easy to germinate) and plant seedlings outdoors after the threat of frost. Dig roots in fall before frost in its first year in cool climates or, in warmer zones, the second fall when the berries are ripe red-orange, and follow the root-processing tips on page 110. I prefer to dry the root, preferably by itself, as its strong scent (its name means "smells like horse") can infiltrate other herbs.

Reishi

Ganoderma lucidum, G. lingzhi, G. tsugae, and other species
Polypore Mushroom

 Appropriate during the daytime. Unlikely to impair function; may have moderately energizing activity.

 Well balanced, with effects that are generally helpful day or night. Unlikely to oversedate by day or overstimulate at night.

Traditional Chinese medicine (TCM) practitioners adore reishi. It's a polypore, which is a mushroom that grows on trees and has pores on its underside. This mild adaptogen-like mushroom calms and strengthens the heart, acts as a lung tonic, and promotes longevity. Its anti-inflammatory and immune-modulating properties make it particularly useful in asthma, allergies, autoimmune diseases, complex postinfection conditions, and cancers. Various reishi species can be used *somewhat* interchangeably. Reishi is too tough to eat and tastes a bit bitter, but it makes excellent medicine.

Mushroom of Immortality

Reishi is one of those "all that and a bag of chips" mushrooms. It offers all the usual medicinal mushroom benefits to strengthen and modulate immune function with complex polysaccharide starches called beta-glucans, yet it also has some bonus superpowers. Reishi calms disturbed "Heart Shen," that is, it tonifies (or restores the vitality of) the physical and emotional heart, improves circulation, nourishes the spirit, quells anxiety, improves sleep, eases fatigue, and restores vitality. Known as the "mushroom of immortality," reishi offers adaptogen-like properties that address stress, as well as gentle energy and longevity.

Reishi reduces inflammation and has been studied in cancer care, asthma, and allergies. Generally it is beneficial in under-functioning immune conditions, as well as autoimmune diseases and complex post-infection states such as chronic Lyme and long COVID. Reishi seems to protect and support the liver. It has a long history of extensive use in Asia. Reishi (as well as the more stimulating chaga and cordyceps) has a strong affinity for the lungs, improving their function and oxygen utilization, making it useful over the long term for people prone to bronchitis and pneumonia, as well as in chronic obstructive pulmonary disease (COPD), fatigue, altitude sickness, shortness of breath, and, once again, long COVID.

Safety and Considerations

Reishi is extremely safe and well tolerated by most. As with most mushrooms, the raw fruiting body should always be cooked or extracted before consumption, though the mycelium is usually safe raw. Reishi is as hard as wood and tastes more bitter than other mushrooms, which makes it more appropriate for medicinal blends than for food-based remedies. Coffeelike flavors, chocolate, molasses, and chai spices make it more palatable. When adding reishi to food, including broth, you may want to limit the quantity for flavor, though larger doses would certainly be safe. Reishi may

have blood-thinning properties, so avoid before surgery and alongside blood-thinning medications. If you're allergic, have difficulty digesting, or are sensitive to mushrooms, you may not tolerate reishi—sometimes the double-extraction tincture is better tolerated in people with mushroom intolerance, but not always.

Working with Reishi

Mushroom medicine–making is a tad different from working with herbs because you need to slowly cook raw fruiting bodies (ideally in hot water) to render them digestible and safe. I highly recommend *Christopher Hobbs's Medicinal Mushrooms: The Essential Guide* to learn more about medicinal mushrooms and remedy-making techniques. Learn how to

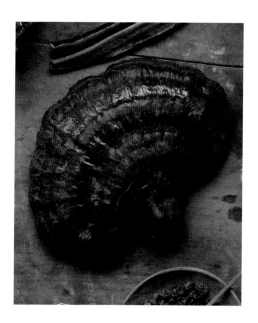

make a double-extraction tincture and concentrated syrup—excellent for reishi—via the book bonus webpage in Resources on page 178.

Part used: mushroom fruiting body (cook first!) or mycelium

Tea or broth decoction: 1–2 slices or more per 16 ounces, simmered 20 minutes or longer

Double-extraction tincture: 1–3 mL, one to three times daily, solo or in formula
    Dried 1:5 in 30 percent alcohol

Mycelium or heat-extracted powder/capsules: 1–6 g per day in capsules or mixed into food—pairs well with molasses, chocolate, coffee, roasted roots, cinnamon, chai spices. Check out Asia Suler's Reishi Maple Truffle recipe online (follow the book bonus link in Resources, page 178).

Recipes: Reishi Chai (variation), page 132 • Adaptogen "Coffee," page 134 • Adaptogen Frozen Iced "Coffee" (variation), page 134

Growing and Harvesting Reishi

The *Ganoderma* genus of tough, woody mushrooms grows on various species of decaying trees. Sometimes called shelf mushrooms, they jut out from trees and logs like little platforms for a frog or woodland fairy to rest upon. Classic reishi species include *G. lucidum*, which prefers hardwoods and is cultivated in China, and hemlock-loving *G. tsugae*, which grows throughout the Northeast and Northwest. Both have a shiny varnished appearance, ranging from orange-brown to maroon. Various *Ganoderma* species and colors, including artist's conk (*G. applanatum*), have similar overall medicinal qualities yet differing tendencies and organ affinities. Cultivate reishi on logs and stumps by drilling holes in the wood and inoculating them with plug or sawdust spawn, making sure to match the species with its preferred tree type. Cut the fruiting body while it's growing—it will have a light yellow/white outer edge. Freeze to kill or manually remove beetle larvae. It is best sliced into thin strips before drying—some species are impossible to process once dried.

Holy Basil (Tulsi)

Ocimum sanctum, syn. *O. tenuiflorum*, and other species
Mint Family (Lamiaceae)

 Well balanced, with effects that are generally helpful day or night. Unlikely to oversedate by day or overstimulate at night.

A delicious, delightful herb, holy basil (also known as tulsi) excels at relaxing the mind and body, improving cognition, and lifting the spirits. It also lowers blood sugar, modulates cortisol, decreases inflammation, enhances digestion, and strengthens the immune system. It is among my favorite herbs to address the sleep–stress connection. Several species and varieties are used somewhat interchangeably. I most often work with "temperate" tulsi, recently recognized to be an *O. africanum* variety, because it's easy to grow abundantly in most gardens and makes swoon-worthy medicine when used fresh or freshly dried.

Calm Energy Zen

Inhaling and consuming this herb evokes the Zen-like quality of meditation or surrounding yourself with incense. The intense, sweet flavor and hints of clove, mint, fruity bubble gum, and basil aromas create a divine experience as tea, though other forms of medicine also work well. As an adaptogen and nervine, holy basil both calms and energizes the spirit, quells anxiety and grief, and brings clarity and focus to the mind. As a cortisol modulator, it not only eases stress but also reduces blood sugar, bad cholesterol, triglycerides, and sugar cravings (especially stress-induced!). Consider it throughout the day or after dinner to relax. It blends well with relaxing, restorative herbs including oat, rose, and lemon balm as well as adaptogens.

Great Protector

Tulsi is associated with the Hindu god Vishnu and is used for medicinal protection in Ayurveda. The holy basil group of plants

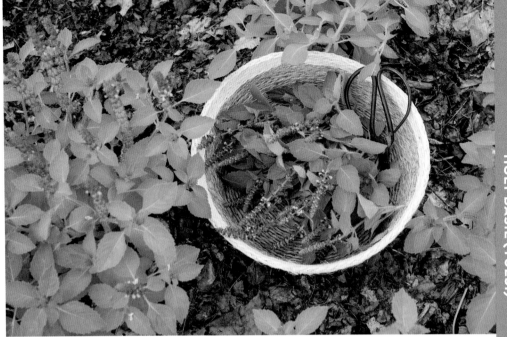

Pots of tulsi often adorn Hindu temples, creating sacred space and bringing prayers to heaven with its calming aroma. This "temperate" or Kapoor tulsi is my favorite to grow.

have traditionally been enjoyed throughout Southeast Asia, Africa, and Latin America. Holy basil fortifies the immune system to fight infections, modulates overreactive immune responses, increases digestive function and juices, and protects against ulcers and radiation. It may stimulate anti-cancer activity and fights both oxidative stress and inflammation with its antioxidant and anti-inflammatory properties. Holy basil makes its way into formulas for almost every body system or health concern—it's that kind of plant. As an anti-inflammatory COX-2 inhibitor, it helps fight many chronic diseases and eases pain, especially when combined with other anti-inflammatory herbs like turmeric, ginger, rosemary, or ashwagandha.

Safety and Considerations

Holy basil is safe for adults and children and usually does not interact with medications. Some may find its digestive effects too stimulating. Because holy basil (particularly unsweetened) lowers blood sugar, be careful introducing it in diabetes or alongside blood sugar medications. If you're prone to hypoglycemia, take it with meals or lightly sweetened with honey, go slow, and monitor your glucose levels. In *rare* cases, people feel spacy, anxious, "high," too energized to sleep, or simply don't like holy basil—some of which may relate to its hypoglycemic effects as well as the airy aromatics. It's generally not recommended in pregnancy.

Working with Tulsi

Holy basil comes in many different varieties and species that are somewhat interchangeable. The multiple common and Latin names may be labeled inconsistently in the market—see "Growing and Harvesting Holy Basil" on page 39 for details. Enjoy fresh or freshly dried. Homegrown/dried or direct from the farm will be vastly superior to the bland dried herb dust commonly sold by big international bulk suppliers. Good-quality holy basil is amazing and delightful in any form! Making the hydrosol is an otherworldly experience.

Part used: aerial parts, leaves and flowers

Tea: 1–2 heaping teaspoons dried herb/cup, infusion, 1–3 cups daily

Tincture: 1–3 mL, one to three times daily, solo or in formula

Fresh 1:2 in 95 percent alcohol (best) or dried 1:5 in 50–60 percent alcohol

Honey, oxymel, glycerite, syrup: 1 teaspoon as needed (heavenly!)

Capsules/powder: 500–2,000 mg crude herb daily

Other uses: cordial, infused water, seltzer/soda, hydrosol, bath

Recipes: Maria's Sleep Tea (variation), page 123 • Holy Rose Water, page 124 • Other Holy Basil Beverages, page 124 • Stress Relief Tincture Blend, page 148 • Mellow Me Glycerite, page 152 • Herbal Sleep Pillow, page 159

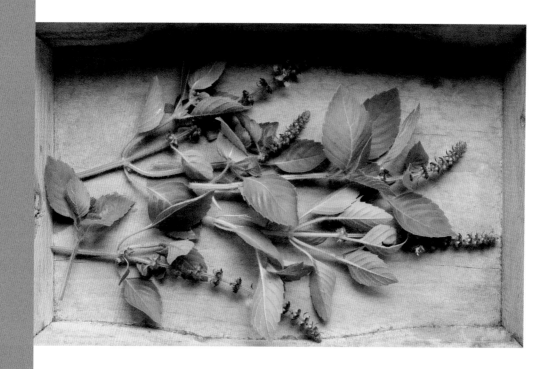

Growing and Harvesting Holy Basil

Like its fellow basils, tulsi is an annual that jumps for joy when everything else in your garden bows in submission to hot-as-Hades midsummer temps, and begins rapidly producing abundant medicine—provided you've given it rich and moist yet well-drained garden soil. It detests cool temps and dies at the kiss of frost.

What Kind of Holy Basil?

There are several varieties to choose from that are somewhat interchangeable medicinally, and often labeled inconsistently in the market. You'll see all of them listed as holy basil, sacred basil, or tulsi.

- *Ocimum sanctum* (recently renamed *O. tenuiflorum*); varieties include 'Rama', 'Krishna', 'Amrita'

- Kapoor, the "temperate tulsi"—now recognized as a variety of *O. africanum*—is the most commonly sold type of holy basil grown in North America.

- *Ocimum gratissimum*, also known as Vana tulsi

If you want to geek out over the subtle differences of the different species and varieties, see the writings of Richo Cech and the University of Georgia study published by Noelle Fuller online. If your seed catalog offers one type and does not specify the variety, it's probably temperate tulsi, which grows most abundantly in temperate climates and may also self-seed. Temperate tulsi is what I prefer to grow and work with. Some tulsi types are perennial in warm zones or if brought indoors. Temperate tulsi produces nonstop flowers, which you can trim regularly (to enjoy for tea, water, medicine) to encourage growth. At first, simply pinch off tulsi's flowers. Once it's bushy and vibrant, later in the season, trim the top one-half to two-thirds.

Magnolia

Magnolia species
Magnolia Family (Magnoliaceae)

 Well balanced, with effects that are generally helpful day or night. Unlikely to oversedate by day or overstimulate at night.

 Appropriate at night. Unlikely to keep someone awake with stimulating properties; may be more strongly sedating.

The graceful magnolia tree you admire in landscapes and city parks holds more value for medicine and sleep than you may realize. The bark smells and tastes delightful—like lemongrass and root beer—and the tincture is one of my favorite ingredients in sleep and daytime blends to modulate dysregulated stress hormones that cause people to wake in alarm mode at 2 a.m. Magnolia gently supports the nervous system with adaptogen-like, nervine, and calmative qualities.

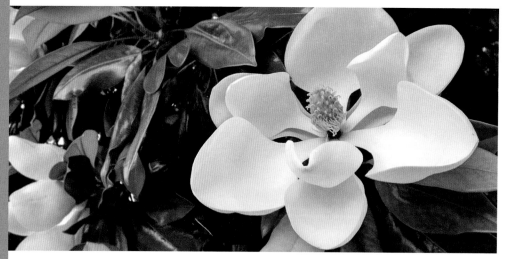

Many people grow this gorgeous landscape tree without realizing its many medicinal virtues.

Adaptogens for Sleep Support

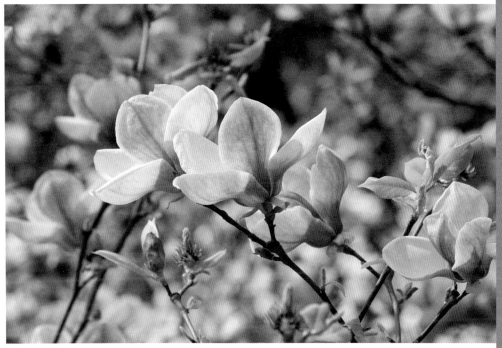

Adrenals, Stress, and Sleep

Magnolia bark modulates and reduces the stress hormone cortisol. Naturopath Mary Bove taught me to turn to magnolia to help people who can't sleep due to stress and cortisol imbalance, especially those who wake in the middle of the night and can't fall back to sleep. Studies show that alkaloids in the bark increase relaxation, decrease the length of time to fall asleep, and increase both REM and non-REM sleep for more restorative slumber. Magnolia also eases anxiety, mild depression, and menopause symptoms and improves weight management when stress is a factor. It's fabulous in blends with adaptogen, nervine, antidepressant, or sedating herbs, as well as herbs for hormone or blood sugar balance, day or night.

A Long History throughout Asia

Traditional Chinese and Japanese Kampo practitioners love magnolia and work with it in very diverse ways. They employ the flowers to disperse and clear heat and the bark to regulate qi (life force) and reduce stagnation. Studies support its anti-inflammatory and immune-supportive effects with a history of use for malaria arthritis; modern herbalists including

Debbie Mercier incorporate it in Lyme coinfection protocols. Consider magnolia as a subtle pain-nervine remedy, also useful in joint inflammation and rheumatoid arthritis.

Safety and Considerations

It appears safe, though little modern scientific data is available.

Working with Magnolia

Best fresh or freshly dried. The beneficial alkaloids are not very water soluble. Though popular in traditional Chinese medicine and a common landscape tree, magnolia is tricky to find commercially fresh or freshly dried. It's available in pill form and a few commercial sleep blends. Some small-scale herbalists sell it solo dried or tinctured.

Part used: bark (stronger), flowers

Tincture: 1–3 mL, one to three times daily, solo or in formula

Fresh 1:2 in 95 percent alcohol (best) or dried 1:5 in 50–60 percent alcohol

Recipe: Maria's Go-To Sleep Tincture Blend, page 146 • Stress Relief Tincture Blend (variation), page 148

Growing and Harvesting Magnolia

Magnolia is a popular landscape tree (hardy in USDA Zones 4–10). *Magnolia officinalis* is the official species used as medicine in Asia (where it is native), but all species can be used relatively interchangeably, including the closely related tulip tree (*Liriodendron tulipifera*). I love my star-kobus magnolia hybrid and appreciate herbalist Leslie Williams for teaching me that it's great medicine. Leslie particularly favors the star magnolias for sleep. Different species vary in strength. The best magnolias have a pleasant, strong aroma and flavor when you scratch the bark, reminiscent of root beer and lemongrass. The strength of the aroma and flavor is an indicator of the plant's potency. Prune the bark in any time of year or use the freshly opened flowers, which are not quite as strong as the bark. I particularly enjoy the juicy bark of new growth in late summer.

Additional Adaptogens to Consider

The above adaptogens and adaptogen-like herbs are among my favorites to support day-time stress levels while also supporting sleep, particularly if well matched to the person and taken on a regular basis. They're also the most sustainable and easily available commercially or to grow or wildcraft. However, the following adaptogens may also be helpful.

Shatavari (*Asparagus racemosus*)

This Ayurvedic herb from India is some-times called "the herb of 100 uses" and the herb for "the woman with 100 husbands." As you might expect from such a name, this is a multifaceted herb with queenlike energy that has a particular affinity for juicy estrogen balance for people deal-ing with PMS, fertility issues, peri- and postmenopause—though everyone can safely consume it. Shatavari moistens tissues and enhances lubrication through-out the body. It is nourishing, restorative, gently calming, and helps soothe dryness, irritation, and inflammation not only in the reproductive organs but also in the urinary and digestive tracts, as well as the joints—particularly supporting tissues that get dry and lax when estrogen wanes.

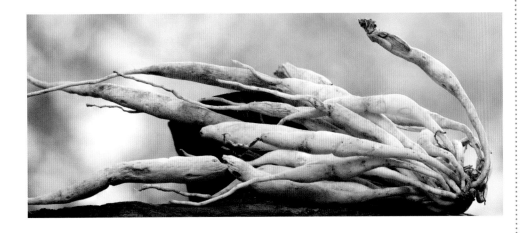

Maca
(*Lepidium meyenii*)

This staple root crop indigenous to the Andes is related to turnips. Maca is rich in protein and minerals if you consume it as a powder, and it provides gently energizing adaptogen activities. Maca is also moistening to tissues, boosts libido and mood, and seems to support testosterone, estrogen, and progesterone balance in all genders, including during menopause and andropause. It tastes good—slightly sweet and nutty, like the inside of a malted milk ball. It blends well in food and coffeelike recipes, particularly with cacao. If you don't digest raw turnipy roots well, consider the tincture. Only purchase fair-trade Peruvian-sourced maca, from reputable suppliers, preferably organic.

Schizandra
(*Schisandra chinensis*)

This robust woody vine from traditional Chinese medicine produces tangy little berries that are intensely sour as well as bitter, sweet, salty, and pungent, hence the TCM name *wǔ wèi zi,* which means "five flavor fruit." It's excellent for calm, clarity, focus, energy, and cognition. Some people may find it overstimulating, especially in higher doses. Schizandra also supports liver protection and detoxification but may affect the metabolism of some drugs; it offers additional benefits for deep immune support, fluid balance, enhanced digestion, and overall vitality. I enjoy the complex, tangy berries in sweet-and-sour recipes (such as the tea on page 128), tincture, and glycerite, or you can simply chew a few

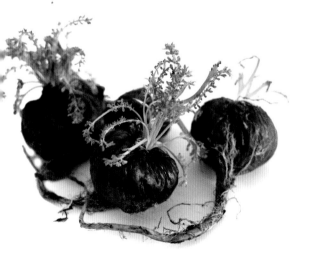

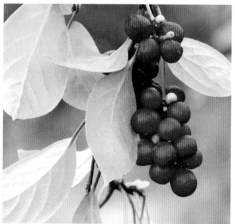

Managing Stress and Daytime Energy

berries with breakfast. It's among the more sustainable and easier-to-grow adaptogens, though it takes several years to bear fruit in abundance. Depending on the variety and species, schizandra may be self-fertile or require both male and female plants to fruit. *Schisandra sphenanthera* is medicinally interchangeable with *S. chinensis*. The vigorous vine growth reminds me of invasive bittersweet; ensure a sturdy trellis system or arbor.

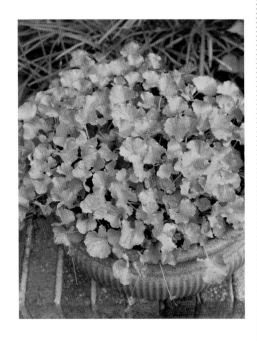

Gotu Kola
(*Centella asiatica*)

This leafy creeping ground cover is the most subtle of the adaptogens—gently and slowly enhancing cognition with mild calming activity over months of regular consumption. It more rapidly supports circulation, vascular health, and the healing of various types of tissues, including nerves, the gut lining, wounds, and collagen. Herbalist David Winston recommends this cooling leafy green when tissue is red, hot, and inflamed. Large doses—an ounce or more per day—will produce better results, but that can be difficult to source. It's easy to grow and is often consumed as a slightly bitter, celery-ish leafy green in tropical climates of Hawaii, India, and Southeast Asia, including Sri Lanka and Vietnam, as well as parts of Africa. Gotu kola prefers super-rich, warm, waterlogged soil. Add it to smoothies, salads, soups, or green juice, or enjoy it in tea and typical remedy formats. It's not delicious, but you can cover it up with other flavors. In Southeast Asia it's consumed as a sweetened pick-me-up drink, and is often called pennywort. (Note that this common name is also used to refer to plants other than *Centella asiatica*.) Though the adaptogenic properties are profound when it is sourced from hot climates, the international herb market quality is often lacking. The best quality tends to come from Sri Lanka and Hawaii, and you can also grow your own anywhere with some TLC.

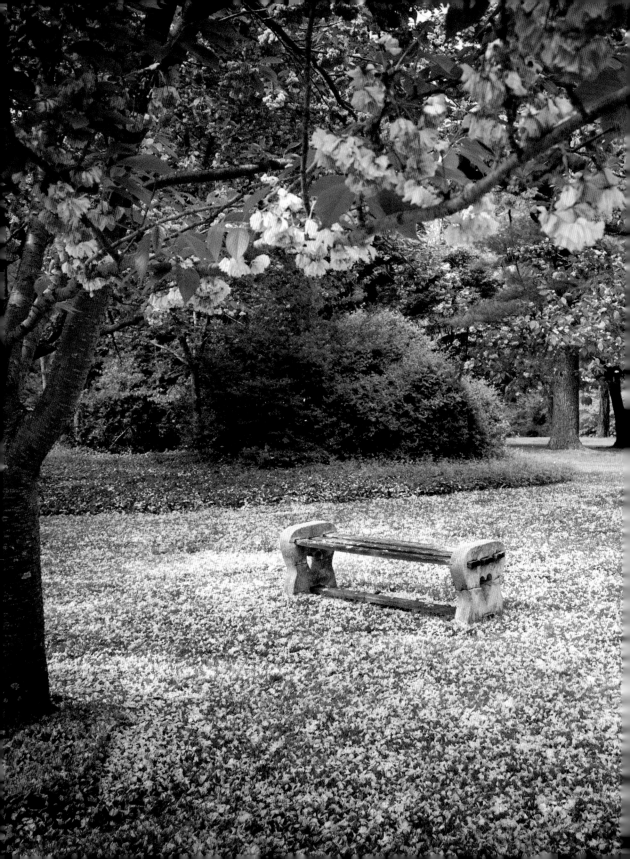

CHAPTER 3

Relaxation Day and Night

When people turn to sleep aids, the first thing they typically reach for—whether herbal or pharmaceutical—is a sedative. It makes sense. We associate sedation with sleep, and when you're not sleeping well, you're desperate for something to "knock you out." However, that's not always the best approach. Certainly, sedative herbs are often helpful for sleep, but it can be even more effective and more broadly beneficial to step back and support relaxation.

Why Relaxation Matters

Many of our everyday health complaints stem from spending too much time in the fight-or-flight mode and not enough in the rest-and-repair mode. Adaptogens (from Chapter 2) are nice, but when you give your body the opportunity to *relax*, it finally has the chance to tend to its maintenance duties, with the following results.

* Better mood and sleep

* Steadier metabolism and blood sugar and insulin curves

* Reduced inflammation

* Improved digestion, absorption of nutrients, and elimination

* Improved immune function

* Increased detoxification via the liver, kidneys, and so forth

* Calmer and stronger cardiovascular system, and decreased blood pressure

Eliciting the relaxation response and bringing the central nervous system down a notch aids a range of common mood and stress issues, including anxiety, panic attacks, focus difficulties, hyperactivity, depression . . . and insomnia.

Supporting our relaxation response throughout the day *and* night helps downregulate the stress hormones and mood imbalances that often trigger insomnia. Relaxing herbs and lifestyle techniques before bedtime give us additional support and may be all we need to shift sleep cycles in our favor. Supporting overall relaxation and a balanced stress response helps us get to the root of our sleep disturbances and overall well-being, rather than simply trying to conk out just before bed. When you ignore the underlying stressors, triggers, and daytime nervous-adrenal patterns, even if sedatives initially seem to help, often the body eventually adapts and sleeplessness returns.

That's not all. Compared to sedatives, herbs and approaches that support overall relaxation also tend to be more safe, appropriate, and free of side effects for a wider range of people. Stronger sedatives may have unwanted side effects depending on the herb and your individual situation. Sedatives may worsen sleep apnea as well as some types of sleep disorders like sleep paralysis. They are more likely to interact negatively with pharmaceuticals that also relax the central nervous system, including most antidepressants, antianxiety medications, and some pain, seizure, and nerve medications. And they may aggravate depression and sluggishness in some people, especially at high or even regular doses. Some people with trauma may find that their bodies resist sedation but feel gently cradled and supported by the more gentle and restorative relaxation approaches, especially over the long term. (We discuss the pros and cons of sedatives further in Chapter 4.)

To quote herbalist jim mcdonald, "Gentle does not mean weak." Our relaxation herbs and approaches offer some immediate benefits and, when employed regularly over the long term, can move mountains.

You Are How You Think and Feel: Mind–Body Balance

A less tangible, but equally important, pillar of health is mind–body balance, or mind–body–spirit balance. Cultivating mind–body balance helps you live in relaxation mode more often and avoid getting stuck in stress mode. How you think and feel has a direct effect on your overall health and vice versa. While taking care of your body via diet, exercise, and reduced toxin exposure will also benefit your mind and spirit, consider giving mind–body wellness some direct TLC. This will specifically help your nervous and endocrine systems and your stress response and augment your resistance to a range of diseases, from mood disorders and heart disease to cancer.

Of course, just telling yourself to be calm, think positively, and stay centered won't always do the trick. Changing your perspective and thinking habits can seem daunting. Fortunately, certain activities directly nourish your mind and spirit to make this transition easier. Bringing some of these tasks into your daily life will slowly and profoundly shift your reality toward one of health and balance.

MEDITATE

Just 8 weeks of mindfulness meditation approximately 30 minutes a day can help you feel calmer and make positive changes in various areas of your brain, including improved memory, empathy, sense of self, and stress regulation. Studies also support meditation's ability to decrease blood pressure, heart disease risk, anxiety, depression, insomnia, and addictive behaviors. Some of the most profound research on meditation is based on mindfulness-based stress reduction techniques and programs. Classes and books will help you get started. Once you have the basics, you can meditate anywhere, even in short bursts.

BREATHE

Sure, you're always breathing. But specific breathwork can help pull you out of the fight-or-flight stress response and into relaxation, and shift your focus inward. Most forms of meditation and yoga incorporate breathwork, but you can also try specific short breathing exercises. One of my favorites is the 4-7-8 breath touted by integrative healing expert Dr. Andrew Weil. In a sitting position, place your tongue gently on the roof of your mouth, by your teeth. Breathe out through your mouth with a "whoosh" sound. Inhale through your nose to the count of four. Hold your breath for the count of seven. Then exhale through your mouth to the count of eight. Practice this breath at least four times in a row, and up to eight times (but no more than that in one sitting). You can do this as often as you'd like throughout the day, but doing it at least once or twice is ideal. Dr. Weil describes it as "water cutting the Grand Canyon." It can single-handedly make profound changes, but it doesn't happen overnight. I once led a multifaceted course on happiness for 50 people through my local

co-op, and this breathing exercise ranked number one among students for helping them feel calmer, happier, and more at peace. To learn more, check out Weil's book *Spontaneous Happiness* and his free video demo online; access it via the link to my online book extras in Resources, page 178.

TRY YOGA, TAI CHI, OR QI GONG

These ancient practices from India and China were developed by masters of mind–body–spirit balance to guide their students to a better state of being. They incorporate gentle movement and breathwork to increase your vital force. They also improve strength, flexibility, and balance.

BE GRATEFUL AND CULTIVATE OPTIMISM

As you will see, little tasks done regularly can accumulate for phenomenal positive changes in your well-being. Gratitude and optimism are key traits that improve your mental and physical health, and they're surprisingly easy to develop. Consider keeping a gratitude journal where you write down three good things that happen to you each day. Research suggests that daily gratitude alone can improve your overall happiness by as much as 25 percent.

Relaxation beyond Herbs

Before we dive into my most beloved herbs, let's remember that you don't *need* to take herbs to elicit your relaxation response. Many lifestyle practices help calm the nervous system—these changes matter *most* for long-term well-being. Herbs do offer fabulous assistance in soothing the neuroendocrine system, flipping the switch so that you feel less stressed and enjoy a better mood, more energy, and better overall health and vitality, but I think of herbs as training wheels and allies we can turn to in times of need. Adopting supportive lifestyle practices is what promotes the deepest, most sustainable changes long term. Choose one or two approaches that feel most enticing, beneficial, and doable for you. These practices may include the following.

* Daily and/or bedtime meditation

* Deep breathing exercises

* Yoga

* Tai chi

* Qi gong

* Exercise (preferably earlier in the day), including even a short walk

* Eating more plants

* Time outdoors in nature

* Walking barefoot on the earth

* Gardening

* Art therapy, doodling, music, dancing, or journaling

* Gratitude exercises

* Laughter

* Aromatherapy

* Taking a bath

* Scheduling massage or energy work—or trading with loved ones

* Therapy such as cognitive-behavioral therapy or trauma work

* Restructuring your life, saying no when you need to, valuing your well-being, letting go of that which does not serve you, and reducing exposure to potentially toxic relationships

* Scheduling personal time for self-care

* Creating clearer boundaries for work, screen time, and so forth

* Long hugs and snuggles with loved ones, animals, or trees

Baby steps are okay and often more realistic! Start with a tip or two that is most appealing, easiest, and impactful for you. Understand that life is full of ebb and flow—perfection isn't the goal. I suggest pairing relaxing herbs with one or two relaxing lifestyle changes, which will help you start your relaxation journey.

The Power of Daily Tea

Regardless of plant chemistry, just sipping a cup of tea can have therapeutic effects: Studies show that holding a warm cup in your hands encourages warmth and kindness to others and helps you perceive others in a better light. (It's true—a warm drink makes you a nicer person!) It's also interesting to note that many of the herbs that benefit our nervous system—particularly the relaxing ones—are highly aromatic, so that a cup of tea provides not only the healing constituents you swallow but also the vapors you inhale. The beauty of flowers and garnish in your drink relax and lift your mood, like a bouquet of cut flowers does. For these reasons, a daily tea ritual is one of the best ways to allow herbs to multitask and help you feel better. Whether you're sitting in a comfy chair, at the dinner table, in the garden, or even in your car on the way to work, sipping a calming brew tends to your nervous system on many levels. The simple act of making and drinking tea is an affirmation that you are taking care of yourself and that plants—and your body—have the power to heal.

That said, a big cup of tea right before bed might disrupt sleep by making you need to get up and pee. Brew pre-bedtime teas small and strong. Some herbs also taste better as tea (holy basil and lemon balm!), while others like hops, motherwort, and valerian are vile for most taste buds. Tinctures and capsules may be more convenient or palatable for you. You can also try more creative options such as mixing herbal powders into smoothies, ghee, warm milk, or honey.

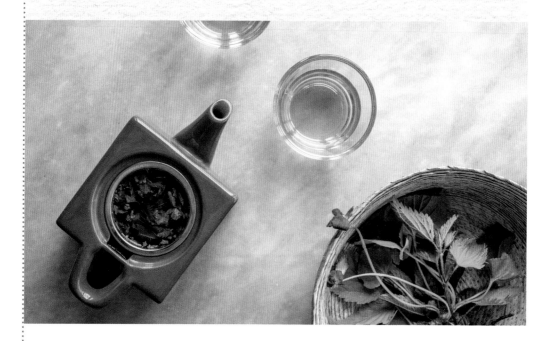

GENTLY CALMING AND UPLIFTING NERVINES

Adaptogens and sedatives get all the attention in product marketing, but nervines are often our greatest allies for stress, sleep, and anxiety.

What's a nervine? *Some* herbalists use the term to refer to any herb that affects the nervous system in any way, including strong stimulants and sedatives. But I use the term the way most of my colleagues do: specifically for restorative herbs that nourish and rebuild vitality and resiliency in the nervous system to promote nervous-adrenal system well-being.

Restorative nervines have a calming effect but are not usually strongly sedating. They support the parasympathetic nervous system's "relaxation response," which is the mode we're supposed to be in most of the day. They're generally helpful throughout the day to calm frayed nerves without making you sleepy or sluggish—an important benefit for those of us who have things to get done during the day! Yet the relaxing effects also help you unwind at night, enhancing sleep when taken before bedtime. Many nervines also uplift mood.

Nervines are appropriate for almost anyone and are unlikely to aggravate gloomy depression, sleep apnea, or sleep disorders, or interact with medications; stronger sedatives might aggravate or interact with these. Nervines blend well with adaptogens or sedatives in formula if you'd like to pep up or bring things down a notch. Let's explore some of my favorites.

Be sure to see the tips for taking herbs in Chapter 6, page 118, and for additional safety tips, including for people taking medications, for children, in pregnancy, and during lactation, see Chapter 7.

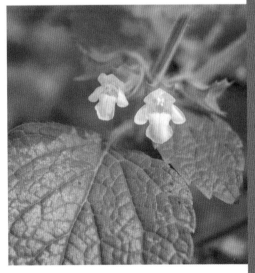

High-quality fresh lemon balm extract is a fantastic nervine for sleep and daytime calm.

Milky Oat Seed

Avena sativa
Grain/Grass Family (Poaceae)

 Well balanced, with effects that are generally helpful day or night.
Unlikely to oversedate by day or overstimulate at night.

All parts of the oat plant, a member of the grain family, are nutritious and gently calm the nervous system. However, the fresh milky oat seed most specifically offers unique benefits from special compounds that soothe, calm, rebuild, and nourish your nervous-adrenal system while quelling agitation. Think of it like food for your nerves.

When You're Wired and Tired

Consider milky oat seed extract during times of depletion and overstimulation: when you feel stress, anxiety, overwork, and adrenal fatigue, or are experiencing attention deficit, hyperactivity, post-trauma, all-nighters, coffee-slugging cubicle work, and harried road trips. It's specifically indicated for when you feel burnt out, wired, and tired, and it combines well in blends. It quells that obnoxious buzzing feeling. Enjoy milky oat solo or blend with adaptogens, nervines, or calmatives such as lemon balm, motherwort, holy basil, ashwagandha, or bacopa. Its flavor is mellow, haylike, and slightly sweet.

Slowly Nourishes and Restores

Milky oat seed slowly builds in its effect—take it in regular, moderately high doses for months or longer to get the best results. Both oat straw and dry milky oat tops lack the overt nervine chemistry of fresh milky oat seed, but they're still a nice nutritive, rich in many supportive minerals. Both the dried tops and straw play a supportive role in nerve-soothing tea infusions and decoctions. As a flower essence, oat helps restless souls convert tentative ideas into direction and find a meaningful path in life.

Gently Calming and Uplifting Nervines

Safety and Considerations

Extremely safe for almost anyone, including kids. Gluten contamination (though unlikely) is possible due to sharing processing equipment with other grains—if you're not growing your own, ask your supplier about cross-contamination potential. Unless contaminated, oats do not contain gluten, and most people with celiac and other gluten sensitivities tolerate oats. However, some people react to the closely related protein avenin. If you know oatmeal disagrees with you, skip all forms of oat.

Working with Oats

Milky oat seed is most potent *fresh* extracted in alcohol for its nervine properties, though other solvents may work. Once dried, oat tops are more like oat straw—primarily nutritious, though taking high doses over the long term can also be nourishing for the nerves. Good-quality milky oat seed, tops, and oat straw are light green, not beige or brown.

Tea (oat straw or dry tops): 1–2 heaping teaspoons to ¼ ounce dried herb/cup; infusion, super infusion, or decoction, 1–4 cups daily; nice in super infusions as well as simmering broths

Tincture (fresh milky seed): 2–5 mL, one to three times daily, solo or in formula

Fresh 1:2 in 95 percent alcohol (best) or vinegar (good) or glycerine (tasty but most likely to get funky over time)—whir in a blender for the best liquid extract

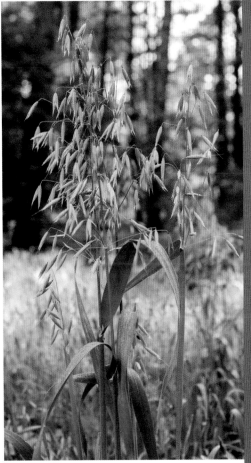

Milky oat seeds are ready only for a few days of the year. White "milk" should spurt out when you squish and pop the fresh seeds.

Ice cubes: whir water and fresh milky oats in a blender, freeze in ice cube trays, and add to tea blends as desired

Recipes: Ashwagandha Chai (variation), page 132 • Stress Relief Tincture Blend, page 148 • Mellow Me Glycerite, page 152

Growing and Harvesting Milky Oats

Oats are a common organic cover crop that offer three forms of herbal medicine—grain, milky oat seed, and straw—each with different applications, yet sharing the same general ability to nourish and soothe. People rarely grow oats in the garden other than as a cover crop. This annual plant prefers full sun and a modest amount of water.

Consider growing oats in a new or old garden bed, or behind shorter plants in the landscape. After the threat of frost has passed in spring, rough up the soil surface, and thickly scatter the seeds. (I use a 5-pound bag for the previous year's 25-by-25-foot chicken run.) Tamp them in lightly. Water periodically if you don't have regular rainfall. Oats will die off in winter and enrich the soil.

Harvesting milky oat seed: Squeeze a few to ensure your plot is ready—they should pop and exude a white "milk." Run your hands up each stalk so the seeds slide off between your fingers, or use a chamomile or blueberry rake. To extract the seeds, whir them in a blender with alcohol, vinegar, glycerine, or water—the blender helps extract more of the good stuff than you can get by simply shoving them in a jar and covering with solvent. Best to use fresh for the nervine properties.

Harvesting oat straw: When the plant is vital, green, and happy (perhaps directly after you harvest the milky seeds), cut one-third to two-thirds of the grassy tops. Dry them. Then use sharp, sturdy scissors to chop them into pieces. Extract vastly more minerals by simmering or making a super infusion.

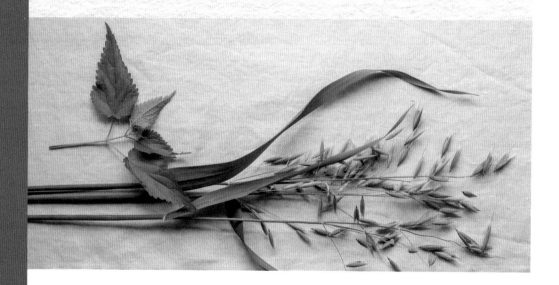

Gently Calming and Uplifting Nervines

Lemon Balm

Melissa officinalis
Mint Family (Lamiaceae)

 Well balanced, with effects that are generally helpful day or night. Unlikely to oversedate by day or overstimulate at night.

 Appropriate at night. Unlikely to keep someone awake with stimulating properties; may be more strongly sedating.

Some of our oldest written herbals extol the many virtues of lemon balm, including Dioscorides's *De Materia Medica* and Ibn Sina (Avicenna)'s *The Canon of Medicine*, and lemon balm is among my most beloved herbs in the clinic. Uplifting, cognition-enhancing, and mildly relaxing, lemon balm can be enjoyed day or night. Studies show it improves calm and cognition within just 1 hour, and offers deeper benefits with regular use. Lemon balm emits a strong "Lemon Pledge" aroma that quickly dissipates once dried—freshness is essential for potency. Lemon balm is lovely solo yet also blends well with other herbs in formula.

Uplifting Calming Nervine

Herbalists prize lemon balm for support of the nervous system; it calms anxiety and aids sleep without oversedating. The lemony aromatics lift the spirit, ease mild to moderate depression (especially in combination with St. John's wort, mimosa, or holy basil), gladden the heart, and quell stress-related benign heart palpitations. For people prone to insomnia, nightmares, anxiety, agitation, frustration, overwhelm, hyperactivity, and/or hypervigilance, consider a cup of lemon balm and holy basil tea (lightly sweetened with honey, if desired) or fresh homemade tincture.

And So Much More

Much like tulsi, lemon balm offers a wide range of benefits with its humble yet tasty leaves. Though best known for the nervous

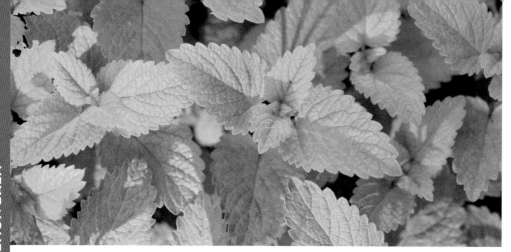

Lemon balm easily tops my list of favorite garden herbs. You can't help but rub its leaves and inhale the spirit-lifting lemon aroma as you walk by.

system, it also supports digestion, viral resilience, healthy inflammatory response, and cardiometabolic health. Lemon balm's aromatic, carminative, and mild bitter properties gently ease digestive distress and improve digestive function and nervous digestion. It also mildly improves blood sugar and heart health. The essential oil and tannins have direct antiviral action when applied topically or taken internally; in the case of herpes, lemon balm may help block the herpes virus out of cells, particularly in the earliest stages of an outbreak. Try dabbing some tincture on contact and taking more internally. Internally, lemon balm may also support people dealing with Epstein-Barr virus, the flu, and early stages of COVID-19. It may help modulate autoimmune disease dysregulation. It's well researched for its ability to improve calm focus and cognitive abilities in all ages, improving levels of the important neurotransmitter acetylcholine, boosting

memory and cognitive skills, and quelling agitation and hyperactivity. As a flower essence (see page 154), lemon balm relaxes and restores, especially during headaches or when you feel your inner resources have been stretched too thin.

Safety and Considerations

Lemon balm is very safe for children, animals, and adults and, in modest amounts, during pregnancy. Very rarely, sensitive people might find it a tad too astringent or stimulating for digestion (leading to stomach upset, nausea), or it may cause hypoglycemia—especially if taken as a strong tea on an empty stomach. A little honey, a shorter steep, the addition of other herbs, or taking it with food helps. Even though it may support people in hyperthyroid states (though rarely sufficient in and of itself to manage this life-threatening disease), it's unlikely to be a problem in hypothyroid disease.

Gently Calming and Uplifting Nervines

Working with Lemon Balm

Use fresh (best) or freshly dried for potency. Lemon balm loses its oomph very quickly once dried. Even the tincture is best within 1 to 3 years. Commercial quality of both tinctures and dry herb tends to be dismal, leading to less impressive effects—grow your own to enjoy fresh or dry at home for tea, or buy freshly dried or tinctured direct from a high-quality farm.

Part used: aerial/leaves

Tea: 1–2 heaping teaspoons dried herb/cup, infusion, 1–3 cups daily

Tincture: 1–5 mL, one to three times daily, solo or in formula

    Fresh 1:2 in 95 percent alcohol

Glycerite, honey, syrup, vinegar: 1 teaspoon as needed

Capsules/powder: 500–3,000 mg crude herb daily

Food: add fresh to pesto, infused water, cordials, smoothies, cake, and other recipes

Aromatherapy: hydrosol, bath, essential oil (expensive!)

Recipes: Maria's Sleep Tea, page 123 • Other Holy Basil Beverages, page 124 • Happy Lemon Tea, page 126 • Chamomile-Mint Tea (variation), page 127 • Lemon Bliss Seltzer, page 130 • Maria's Go-To Sleep Tincture Blend (variation), page 146 • Relief Tincture Blend, page 147 • Stress Relief Tincture Blend, page 148 • Hops Citrus Nightcap Bitters, page 149 • Mellow Me Glycerite, page 152 • Lemon Balm–Catnip Glycerite, page 153

Growing and Harvesting Lemon Balm

This robust perennial (hardy in USDA Zones 4–9) is among our easiest and most abundant herbs to grow! Lemon balm hails from the Mediterranean and will grow almost anywhere, but thrives in moist, well-drained rich soil and dappled sunlight. It spreads by underground root runners and occasionally self-seeds. Cold winters with exposed soil may kill plants but also increase self-seed germination. It may get rambunctious in its favorite spots, but it is not as invasive as spearmint and apple mint. It propagates well from root division. It's tricky to grow in containers but tolerates a big pot with rich soil, good drainage, and careful attention to moisture and warmth. Best harvested before it flowers, especially if you plan to dry it. If it's looking cranky or buggy, cut it back and watch it reemerge vivaciously.

    In fact, lemon balm thrives with several heavy haircuts throughout the season. Handle cuttings gently and dry them with ample airflow and low or no heat to maintain optimal color and flavor—the plant bruises easily with excessive cold, heat, moisture, or mishandling, and the aromas are delicate and easily lost. Harvest aerial parts, preferably before it flowers, several times throughout the season. Use fresh (best) or freshly dried for potency.

Mimosa

Albizia julibrissin
Legume Family (Fabaceae)

 Appropriate during the daytime. Unlikely to impair function; may have moderately energizing activity.

 Well balanced, with effects that are generally helpful day or night. Unlikely to oversedate by day or overstimulate at night.

The mimosa tree—also called albizia and silk tree—doesn't get enough credit in Western herbal medicine even though it grows easily (sometimes too easily . . . it's often invasive) across most of the United States. It's one of our *best* herbs to help lift depression, inspire happiness, and calm and nourish the nervous system.

Tree of Collective Happiness

True to its "collective happiness" name in traditional Chinese medicine, mimosa may be the most broadly helpful, safe, fastest-acting herb to lift the spirits and ease depression, grief, and emotional tension. Research on it is slim—preliminary lab and animal studies confirm antianxiety effects—but it has a long history in TCM. Introduced to the southern United States long ago as a graceful ornamental tree, its medicinal benefits are being disseminated today by herbalists David Winston and Michael Tierra. As a flower essence (see page 154),

mimosa improves intuition, understanding, and sensitivity.

Safety and Considerations

Mimosa has a long history of use in China and appears to be safe for most people. Don't take during pregnancy without supervision. Mimosa may bring trauma to the surface, which often assists trauma resolution but can be unpleasant in the moment if you're not ready. Trauma survivors may want extra support when they first take mimosa, such as before a therapy session. Mimosa may aggravate mania in people

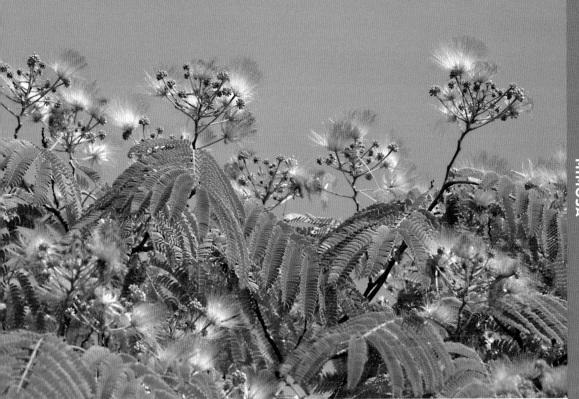

This stunning "tree of collective happiness" from Asia grows quickly into a graceful medium-size tree with fragrant powder-puff pink blossoms.

with bipolar tendencies. Little modern data exists to determine whether it's safe alongside medications, including antidepressants and sedatives, so use caution. That said, herbal clinicians report that mimosa is helpful when clients work with their doctors to wean down antidepressants. *Never* stop or adjust medications without working with your doctor and *slowly* weaning. For more on medications and herbs, see page 166.

Working with Mimosa

Mimosa is difficult to find commercially outside of a few tincture companies that label it as "albizia" and from TCM suppliers, but it's a rampant wild weed tree and ornamental in many ecosystems.

Part used: bark (strongest), flowers

Tea: 1 heaping teaspoon dried herb/cup, infusion, 1–3 cups daily

Tincture, glycerite: 1–5 mL, one to three times daily, solo or in formula

Fresh 1:2 in 95 percent alcohol (best) or (freshly) dried 1:5 in 50–60 percent alcohol

Recipe: Stress Relief Tincture Blend (variation), page 148

Growing and Harvesting Mimosa

Mimosa is a stunningly beautiful, sprawling medium-size tree that grows rapidly and is hardy in USDA Zones 6–9. It grows in full to partial sun and is relatively drought tolerant. Check its status in your state and avoid planting it if it's invasive in your area. It sprouts vigorously from seed. Wildcraft where it's overabundant. It's technically illegal to harvest invasive plants; however, as long as you don't inadvertently spread or propagate it, you're unlikely to run into trouble.

Prune and process the bark (see page 109), preferably in spring or fall. Harvest flowers just as they open, taking care to dry them quickly and store carefully to keep them from turning brown. Enjoy fresh or freshly dried. The bark is more potent, but the delightful aromatic flowers have somewhat similar properties.

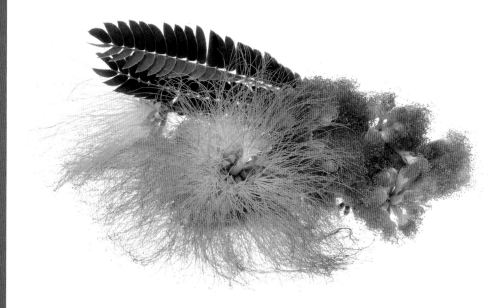

RELAXING NERVINES

These herbs help you get a grip and relax. They're also nervines and still appropriate during the day and in depression (unlike stronger sedatives), but they're more overtly relaxing than the herbs we just discussed. They quickly ground us and bring us back into the "relax, repair, and digest" parasympathetic nervous system. Consider them when your body buzzes with anxiety, agitation, insomnia, or panic and you're feeling excessively sensitive and vulnerable.

The level of sedation depends on the herb, the dose, and your individual response. You might find them perfectly calming during the day, or they may make you want to curl into a ball and go to sleep. You can shift their vibe by blending them with more restorative nervines, gently energizing adaptogens, or stronger sedatives. They can be taken as needed for near-immediate benefit or long term for deeper results.

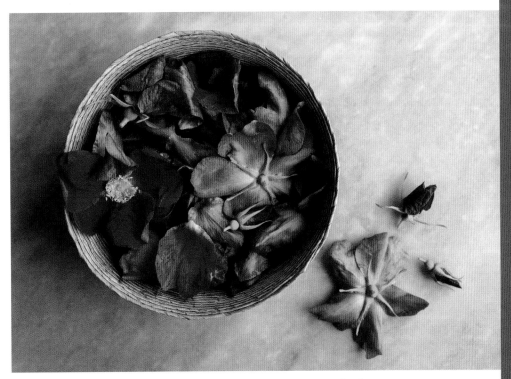

Rose's visual and aromatic presence in remedies evokes peace and calm.

Motherwort

Leonurus cardiaca
Mint Family (Lamiaceae)

 Well balanced, with effects that are generally helpful day or night. Unlikely to oversedate by day or overstimulate at night.

 Appropriate at night. Unlikely to keep someone awake with stimulating properties; may be more strongly sedating.

Motherwort quickly brings down anxiety and panic attacks, particularly if you feel your stress and anxiety in your heart. Its Latin name translates to "lion-hearted," and indeed, motherwort mellows yet brings strength during emotional roller coasters. In spite of its sharp edges and bitter flavor, motherwort softens those who feel overwhelmed, overworked, underappreciated, and on a rampage, as well as during challenging life changes.

Lion-Hearted Mood Care

Motherwort's bitter, grounding energy provides fast relief for anxiety and panic attacks, rivaled only by kava, yet motherwort is safer, easier, and more sustainable to grow. In anxiety and panic, motherwort fosters courage, grounding the nerves and quelling overreactions within 10 to 15 minutes. Taken daily, it takes the edge off worry, frustration, grief, and emotional rampages that occur when you're faced with never-ending demands, a lack of appreciation, and other people's messes. This is particularly helpful for mothers—Rosemary Gladstar says motherwort is for "mothers and people who need a little mothering"—though certainly it supports people of all genders, whether or not they're parents.

I also enjoy motherwort in formulas for depression and a lost spark for life—it blends well with mimosa, holy basil, lemon balm, other nervines, sedatives, and calming adaptogens. It does not appear to interact with antidepressant and antianxiety medications. As a flower essence (page 154) and a tincture, motherwort helps you develop healthy boundaries so you can tend to your *own* care while still being warm and loving with others.

Branching Out

Motherwort also provides "lion-hearted" support for the cardiovascular system, particularly when anxiety and stress manifest as mild chest tightness, hypertension, pings of pain, or palpitations, and it combines well with more overt heart tonics such as hawthorn. But it's not sufficient in acute or life-threatening cardiac states; in those situations seek medical care—conventional medications may also be needed. For the reproductive system, motherwort helps cool hot flashes and mood swings in perimenopause and PMS—particularly when they are exacerbated by stress—and has the potential to induce or increase menstrual flow.

Safety and Considerations

While generally safe, even for children, motherwort's strong bitter flavor makes it undesirable in tea, potentially nauseating in large doses, and less popular for kiddos (try lemon balm or skullcap instead). Though safe while nursing, don't use in pregnancy due to its emmenagogic effect (promoting menstruation). Like lemon

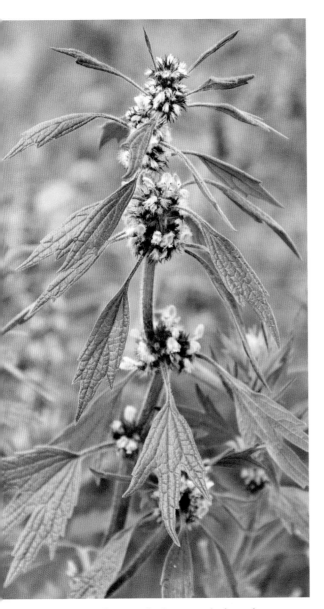

Motherwort looks scraggly, but when you get close up to its beautiful flowers, you'll feel its fierce, loving energy that takes the edge off anxiety and frustration.

balm, even though it may take the edge off hyperthyroid-related agitation, anxiety, and palpitations, it's not sufficient on its own for this potentially lethal disease, and it's usually not a problem in hypothyroid conditions.

Working with Motherwort

Best fresh and tinctured (or try the glycerite, vinegar, or oxymel for an alcohol-free remedy). The tea is unpalatably bitter for most, but some people liken its effects to a warm hug.

Part used: aerial/leaf and flower

Tincture: 1–3 mL, one to three times daily, solo or in formula

Fresh 1:2 in 95 percent alcohol

Glycerite, syrup, vinegar, oxymel: 2–5 mL as needed

Recipes: Maria's Go-To Sleep Tincture Blend (variation), page 146 • Relief Tincture Blend, page 147 • Stress Relief Tincture Blend (variation), page 148 • Hops Citrus Nightcap Bitters (variation), page 149

Growing and Harvesting Motherwort

Tiny, elaborate pink flowers line this spiky, weedy garden herb. It's hardy in USDA Zones 3–9 and does best in rich soil with moderate moisture. When happy, it reaches a robust 5 feet tall. If it's undernourished or dry, it stays spindly, then dies. Motherwort self-seeds rampantly, popping up in new places, which it often prefers. Mine does best in partial shade, but with the right soil conditions, it can thrive in full sun. Harvest aerial parts as it begins to bloom (it goes by quickly!), though you can also harvest it pre-bloom to add to another in-bloom batch. Best in fresh extracts, though you *can* dry it.

Skullcap

Scutellaria lateriflora
Mint Family (Lamiaceae)

 Well balanced, with effects that are generally helpful day or night. Unlikely to oversedate by day or overstimulate at night.

 Appropriate at night. Unlikely to keep someone awake with stimulating properties; may be more strongly sedating.

Think of skullcap when you can't get to sleep or relax because *everything* gets on your nerves—from the stress of the day, a light outside the window, or a worry about tomorrow, to a mosquito flying around the room or your bed partner's obnoxious breathing. Skullcap "caps your skull," nourishes your nerves, and brings your reactions down a notch so you can get some shut-eye. It's specific for those who are overly sensitive, easily irritated by incoming stimuli. Skullcap offers support day and night.

Quell Nerve Irritation and Tension

Skullcap's actions make it helpful not only for insomnia and anxiety but in children and adults alike who have agitation, hyperactivity, and attention-deficit and sensory-processing differences. It works quickly, nourishing and supporting the nervous system, with deeper effects over time. Because it quells nerve irritation *and* relaxes musculoskeletal tension and spasms, it may also help in sciatica, restless legs (when taken along with magnesium and electrolyte support), tension headache, and pain that disrupts sleep. Herbalist Thomas Easley notes that dried skullcap seems more sedating than the fresh plant. Both are lovely when high quality.

Mild Bitter Digestive

Skullcap has a mild bitter flavor with minty undertones and can be employed as a digestive bitter to promote relaxation and aid digestion, especially in nervous bellies. As a flower essence (see page 154), skullcap relaxes and opens the flow of positive energy, particularly between the healer and recipient.

Safety and Considerations

Skullcap is easily identified by its hooded, lipped, unidirectional flowers and their "scutes," dishlike projections on top of their calyxes—yet it's *often* mismarked and adulterated commercially (as well as in many herb books and online photos). Even correctly identified skullcap tends to be low quality when sold commercially, making it best to grow yourself or buy direct from reputable herb farms. True skullcap is quite safe except that it may cause oversedation or aggravate depression and melancholy in rare sensitive people. Be cautious using it alongside sedative and pain medications; it may synergistically oversedate.

Working with Skullcap

Fresh or high-quality dried skullcap works best. Skullcap is often adulterated when sold commercially and is easily mishandled during drying and shipping—even seeds and seedlings may be mislabeled. Grow your own (see the safety tips for ensuring accurate

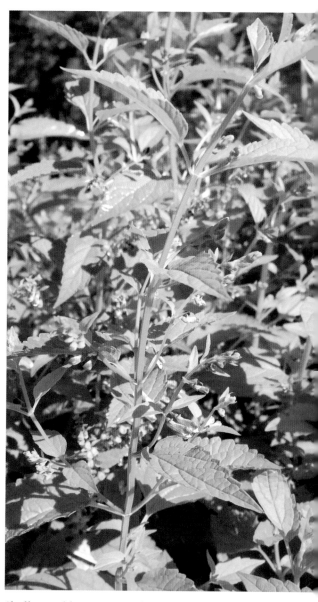

Skullcap sold in stores tends to be low potency and adulterated with liver-toxic germander. Grow your own or buy direct from a reputable farm to ensure quality and identity.

identification), or purchase dried herb direct from trustworthy farms. The few companies I trust for skullcap quality and identity, when I'm purchasing tinctures and dry herb, are listed in Resources on page 178. It's preferable to refresh your tincture supply every 1 to 3 years.

Part used: aerial/leaf, flower

Tea: 1 heaping teaspoon dried herb/cup, infusion, 1–3 cups daily

Tincture: 1–5 mL, one to three times daily, solo or in formula

　　Fresh 1:2 in 95 percent alcohol

Glycerite: ½–1 teaspoon as needed

Topical: bath

Recipes: Maria's Sleep Tea, page 123 • Other Holy Basil Beverages, page 124 • Maria's Go-To Sleep Tincture Blend, page 146 • Stress Relief Tincture Blend (variation), page 148 • Mellow Me Glycerite, page 152

Growing and Harvesting Skullcap

Skullcap is hardy in USDA Zones 4–8. In the wild, you'll find various skullcap species (some of which can be used interchangeably, such as marsh skullcap: *S. galericulata*) growing along the edges of rivers and lakes, often alongside wild mint and bugleweed. In the garden it prefers rich, consistently moist but well-drained soil (particularly in spring), minimal competition, and full to partial sun. It is also finicky in the garden—booming one year, gone or dismal the next. Make plenty of medicine in boom years so you have it during the bust.

　　Harvest happy blooming plants to confirm identity before it goes by. In good years you may get multiple harvests because trimming stimulates new growth. Fresh material works best. If drying, follow the same instructions as for lemon balm—skullcap bruises and loses potency if mishandled. Refresh your tincture supply every 1 to 3 years if possible.

　　Be aware that skullcap seeds and seedlings can be mislabeled (as can photos in herb books and online). Purchase your plants and seeds from reputable sources, wait until the plant flowers, and key it out to ensure you have the right plant—hooded, lipped blue-purple flowers all facing in one direction and a tiny "scute" projection on the calyx, as you can see in the picture and in online articles by herbalist 7Song (available via my book extras web link in Resources, page 178).

Kava

Piper methysticum
Black Pepper Family (Piperaceae)

 Well balanced, with effects that are generally helpful day or night. Unlikely to oversedate by day or over-stimulate at night.

 Appropriate at night. Unlikely to keep someone awake with stimulating properties; may be more strongly sedating.

Kava was one of the first herbs I ever worked with medicinally, back when I was experiencing panic attacks after a traumatic set of events. Alongside doing the deep work to resolve my trauma, kava was an immediate ally to downregulate my anxiety, panic, and tension. It's one of the fastest-acting and most reliable herbs for this, though nowadays I turn more to motherwort, lemon balm, holy basil, and other herbs that are more easily cultivated sustainably in a variety of ecosystems. I prefer reserving kava for acute support as needed.

Numbing Your Tongue and Nerves

Think of kava as your herbal benzodiazepine (like Xanax) for acute anxiety, panic attacks, and hysteria; it acts on similar neurotransmitters, including gamma-aminobutyric acid (GABA), a mood booster and nervous-system relaxant—though thankfully it lacks the drugs' serious side effects and addiction potential. Polynesians traditionally drink kava tea before meetings and celebrations to promote happiness, relaxation, and friendship. It begins working within minutes, and modest amounts are unlikely to interfere with daytime functioning. It has an obvious numbing effect on contact with your tongue, which permeates your body as the medicine kicks in. Kava promotes sleep by relieving anxiety. It has an antispasmodic, analgesic, and numbing

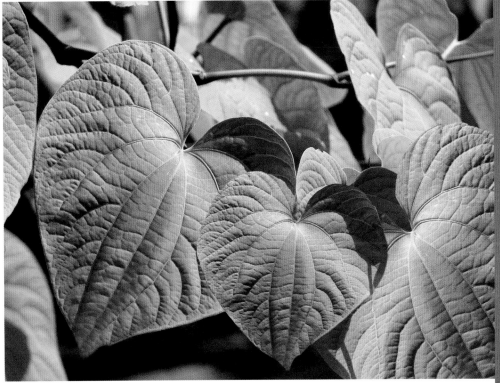

Kava boasts a long history of use throughout the islands of Polynesia to relax and promote friendliness during gatherings and meetings. Inspired by this tradition, kava bars are increasingly popular as a place to unwind without alcohol.

action that decreases pain on contact and can be useful for headaches and genital-urinary-prostate spasms.

Safety and Considerations

Experiencing a numb tongue after drinking kava tea or tincture is normal. Although generally safe with far fewer side effects than its drug counterparts, kava is best used as needed. Consider other herbs for daily support. It's less appropriate for children and may interact with psych and pain medicines as well as alcohol. Kava overuse causes a scaly rash that goes away after stopping use of the herb. Reports of liver toxicity are primarily due to adulteration with aerial parts of the plant. Use only the root, and purchase it only from reputable suppliers. To be on the safe side, avoid kava in cases of liver disease. Avoid the particularly potent and faster-growing Tudei type—it is known to cause nausea and lethargy for 2 days after consumption; this form also seems to be more problematic for the liver than the gentler Noble kava type is.

Working with Kava

Kava isn't typically cultivated outside Polynesia, due to its limited range. The seeds are sterile; kava is typically grown via stem cuttings, which take several years to grow and mature. Ambitious gardeners can do more research and try growing it in a greenhouse. When purchasing kava, seek reputable suppliers and buy the roots whole or cut and sifted. Opt for Noble kava rather than Tudei kava. Grind your kava roots as needed.

Part used: roots

Tea: 1 heaping teaspoon to 2 tablespoons freshly ground roots per 8–16 ounces of hot water. If desired, add a spoonful of coconut oil or milk to increase extraction, steep 10 minutes, then strain (squeezing and kneading the plant material) through a fine-woven cloth.

Tincture: 1–3 mL, one to three times daily, solo or in formula, as needed

Dried 1:5 in 50–60 percent alcohol

Powder/capsules: 1–6 g per day in capsules or mixed into hot milk, ghee, honey, spices

Recipe: Relief Tincture Blend, page 147

Relaxing Nervines

Additional Nervines to Consider

This expansive class of herbs includes many of my favorite plants! Here are a few worthy herbs to consider. You can easily shift the vibe of nervine herbs to be more relaxing or more energizing based on what you pair them with, including adaptogens or sedatives.

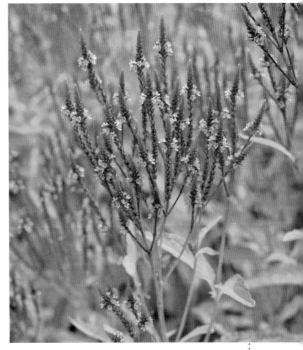

Blue vervain relaxes both physical and emotional tension.

* **Blue vervain** (*Verbena hastata*). This North American native wildflower of waterways is intensely bitter, a flavor that helps bring the nervous system back to the parasympathetic state of relaxation and supports vagal tone and mood. Blue vervain relaxes both physical and emotional tension. Think of it for overscheduled type A control freaks with their shoulders up around their ears, neck and headache pain, and the drive to put everything into lists, Post-it notes, and spreadsheets. (I'm raising my hand here!) It's more about relaxing musculature and tension than sedation; sometimes just a few drops will do the trick. Larger doses are better with food because its intense bitterness can lower blood sugar and stimulate digestion. I enjoy blue vervain as a simple or in blends for people with muscle or nerve pain at night, too. Due to its bitterness, I prefer low doses as tincture. It's great fresh or dried.

* **Wood betony** (*Stachys officinalis*, syn. *Betonica officinalis, Stachys betonica*). This attractive, easy-to-grow garden herb has very similar medicinal actions to blue vervain, yet is more mildly bitter and easier to incorporate into recipes like teas. Many people enjoy the grounding, gently calming, uplifting, antispasmodic activity with additional affinities for headache, backache, and gentle digestive stimulation. It's tricky to find wood betony commercially except from small-scale herb growers

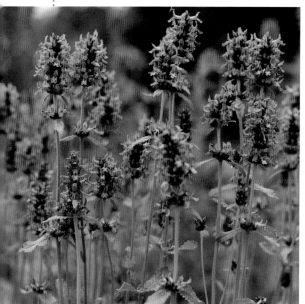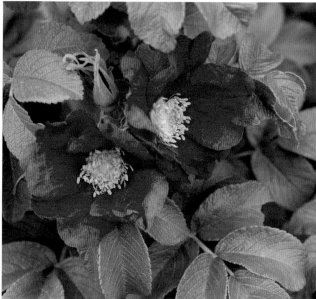

Wood betony and roses offer gentle calming yet uplifting support.

and medicine makers who have come to adore it. Be aware that it shares common names with *Pedicularis* species, which are totally different wild plants, even though some of their pain-related benefits overlap.

* **Roses** (*Rosa* spp.). Any unsprayed wild or heirloom rose with yummy, aromatic flowers can be enjoyed as medicine. Rose gladdens and opens the heart; eases grief, stress, and trauma; and reminds us to "stop and smell the roses" and take time for our own self-care. A fresh flower added to herbal beverages or a sprinkle of dried petals to tea brings a smile every time you smell, see, and sip them. Sweet remedies do a lovely job preserving the aromatics without getting too astringent or bitter—for example, glycerite, infused honey, and so forth. Morning-harvested blooms make a delightful though subtle rosewater hydrosol.

* **Bacopa** (*Bacopa monnieri*). This herb of India and other hot, damp climates is easy to cultivate in similar conditions as gotu kola (page 45). Both herbs are sometimes called "brahmi" and are most famous for supporting cognition, brain, and nerve health. Bacopa supports a calm but not

Relaxation Day and Night

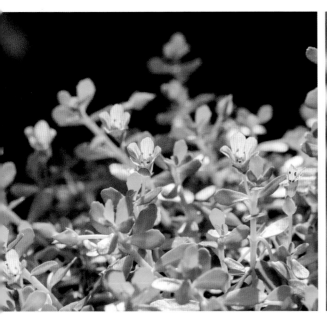
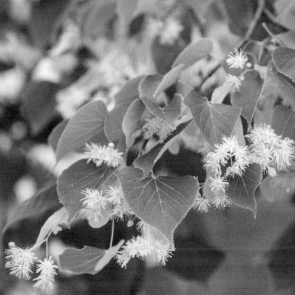

While both bacopa (left) and linden (right) are uplifting, gently calming nervines, bacopa also supports cognition, while linden has an affinity for the heart.

sedated brain state and free memory recall. It's also popular in children's blends for calm, focused attentiveness. But be warned: The flavor is intensely bitter and astringent, like chewing on aspirin or tea leaves. So we often take bacopa as pills, powder, or a tincture and get it over with quickly.

* **Linden** (*Tilia* spp.). This attractive tree with heart-shaped leaves and honey-scented aromatic sweet flowers lines many city streets and parks. It's the inspiration and source of Tilleul in aromatherapy, and is also called lime tree (unrelated to the citrus)

and basswood. The flowers are often sipped in herbal medicine, particularly in Europe, as a relaxing after-dinner tea. Medicinally, linden blossoms offer mild benefits for lowering blood pressure and easing stress and are a welcome addition to any relaxing tea blend. While the leaves are edible, the flowers with the attached leaflike bract are primarily enjoyed for tea and medicine.

* **Damiana** (*Turnera diffusa*, formerly *T. aphrodisiaca*). This aromatic

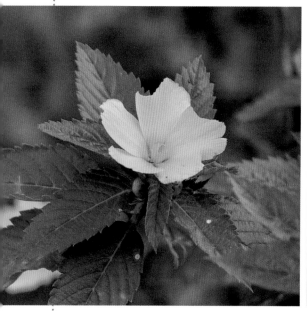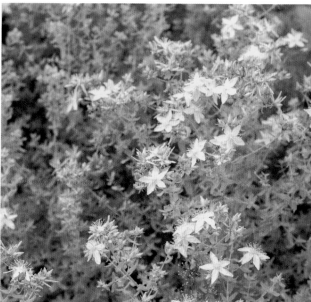

Damiana (left) and St. John's wort (right) uplift the spirits while nourishing the nerves.

flowering shrub grows in the southwest United States, Mexico, Central and South America, and the Caribbean. Throughout this area it is popular for its relaxant, mood-lifting, almost euphoric, and libido-enhancing properties, as well as for balancing the hormones testosterone, estrogen, and progesterone in all genders. The flavor and aroma is intense and a tad unusual, but many people come to adore it.

* **St. John's wort** (*Hypericum perforatum*). The fresh buds and flowers of this sometimes invasive weedy wildflower are well researched and most famous for having benefits in mild to moderate depression, boosting serotonin and other neurotransmitters. That said, it's slow acting and best in steady amounts from a high-quality source—preferably fresh extracted. It offers nervine benefits and isn't as specific for sleep, though some may find it helpful. Topically and internally, it helps soothe and heal agitated nerves, such as in sciatica or after an accident. Unfortunately, ingested St. John's wort interacts with more than half of the medications on the market (more on page 168). I more often turn to mimosa (page 60) to uplift mood, since—at least anecdotally—mimosa

Relaxation Day and Night

is safer alongside medications and typically has faster and more agreeable results.

* **Nutmeg, vanilla, and bay.** These are among the delicious flavors and aromas that offer uplifting, relaxant, nervinelike effects. You don't need much!

* **Magnolia, reishi, ashwagandha, holy basil, shatavari, gotu kola, and schizandra.** These bridge the adaptogen and nervine categories. I really can't overemphasize how valuable these tonic herbs can be for a range of ills. (The term *tonic* refers to generally safe herbs that restore vitality—in this case with an emphasis on nervous-adrenal health, including stress response—and are excellent considerations for daily use.) You can amplify their calming qualities by blending them with other relaxing herbs.

* **Cannabis and hemp.** These—including their isolated cannabinoids (CBD, THC, and others) and aromatic terpenes—have nervine properties, particularly in low doses. See page 104 for more.

* **Flower essences.** These are dilute herbal remedies made with flowers in water, typically preserved with alcohol, that help evoke shifts in our physical, emotional, and spiritual selves. They can also be profound allies solo

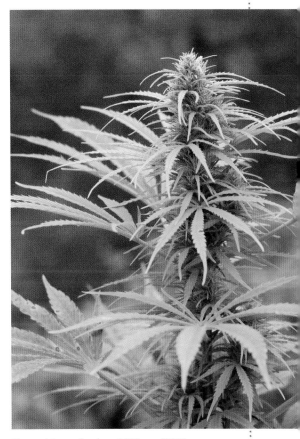

Cannabis—whether CBD- or THC-dominant—may offer nervinelike, calming properties.

or in formulas. Many specific flower essences help us relax, including lavender (spirit calm), valerian (deep peace), and blue vervain (relax control). See page 154 for more on these remedies.

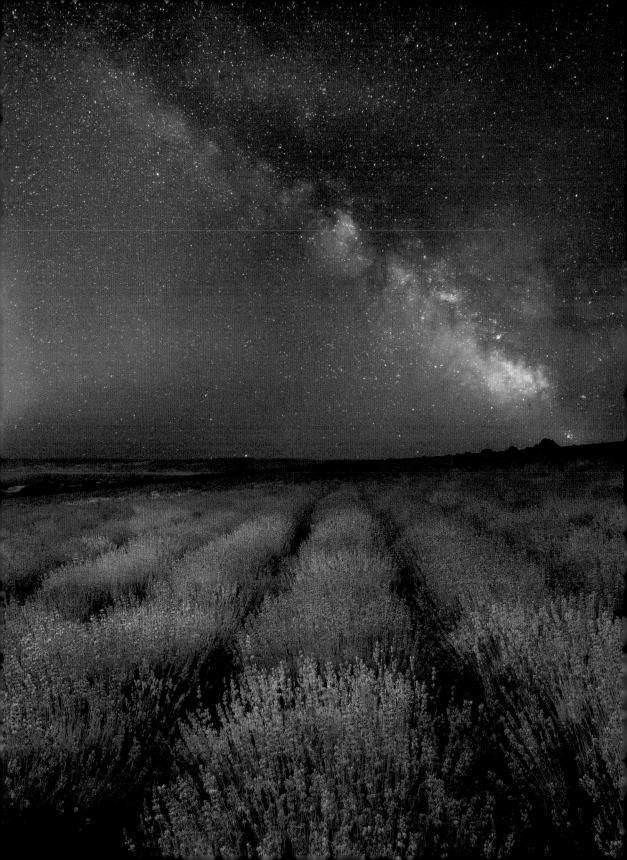

CHAPTER 4

Bedtime Sedating Sleep Support

Perhaps you've just opened this book and skipped ahead to this section, looking for the answers to your sleep difficulties. Although we *will* discuss the classic sleep herbs and important bedtime lifestyle changes in this chapter, I want to call your attention to the prior chapters (particularly Chapter 3, on relaxation) for incredibly useful supports in terms of stress management and relaxation techniques that are helpful day *and* night to promote more restful sleep. In many cases, these herbs and tips are even more helpful and broadly beneficial for more people than the more overt sedative herbs we're about to explore. In addition, Chapter 1 provides important background to help you identify and address your personal insomnia triggers.

With that in mind, we'll now explore the herbs and approaches to try at bedtime to further relax and sedate you to set you up for a better night's sleep.

Before Herbs, Sleep Tips

Herbs are tremendous allies to support sleep, but they're only one small and relatively superficial part of the puzzle. If you haven't read them already—or you need a refresher—check out the tips for regulating sleep cycles by manipulating our relationship with light on page 5 and the core sleep hygiene tips on page 8. These are some of the *most* important tips to improve your sleep tonight and every night going forward.

Herbwise, I love to start with or incorporate into the mix the relaxing herbs discussed in Chapter 3. They often help prepare us for sleep and are less prone to side effects than the more sedating herbs we're about to discuss.

Sedative Herbs for Deeper Relaxation

When the gentle nudge of a nervine or relaxant isn't quite enough, consider sedating herbs. In fact, if you've tried herbs for sleep, chances are sedatives were the first herbs you tried. You may have expected this whole book to be about sedating herbs. Sedatives have a more profound relaxant effect most appropriate at night for sleep, pain, muscular and emotional tension, and anxious states. They can be extremely helpful for sleep, but they're not *always* as broadly beneficial as the nervines we discussed earlier.

In terms of biochemical effects, sedative herbs don't simply put us in the "relaxation response" parasympathetic mode; they actually have an inhibitory or sedating effect on the central nervous system (CNS). Much like sleep and anxiety pharmaceuticals including benzodiazepines (such as Xanax), sedative herbs appear to interact with the neurotransmitter GABA or its receptors, slowing you down and putting you to sleeeeeep. Unlike the benzodiazepine drugs, the herbs are gentler and more nuanced, much safer, and nonaddictive.

CAUTIONS

Because these herbs are stronger on the relaxing spectrum than all the other herbs discussed in this book, they're also less appropriate for some people and in certain situations. Downregulating the CNS could be good or bad: If you weren't quite calm or sleeping well enough, perhaps that extra nudge is just what you

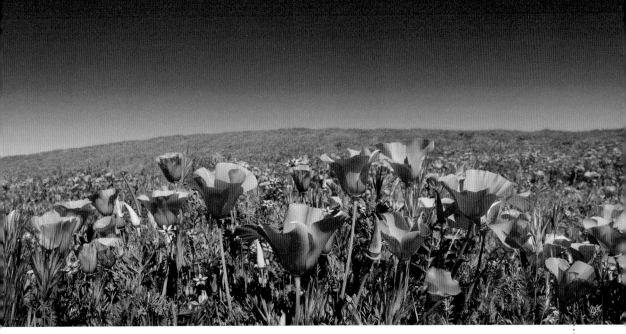

Fields of golden California poppies can be seen across the Southwest. The whole plant provides moderate sedation and pain relief.

need. But oversedating the nervous system can have its downsides if the herb is too strong for you, you take too high of a dose, you take it during the day, and/or you combine it with other CNS sedatives such as alcohol or medications. Many medications are CNS sedatives, including sleep and anxiety medications, most antidepressants, and some pain and nerve medications. If you decide to add these herbs alongside the medications, double-check with your doctor and pharmacist, then introduce herbs gradually, observing to ensure you don't react negatively, and consider enlisting the support of an herbal practitioner for guidance.

What might happen? Sedatives and sedative synergy have the potential to depress the respiratory response, making it harder to breathe, affecting your ability to wake up if you stop breathing due to sleep apnea—which is a problem, because your body needs oxygen. People with certain sleep disorders such as sleep paralysis may find that sedatives make them feel worse. If you're driving or operating heavy machinery at the same time as taking sedative herbs (especially if you combine them with alcohol or sedative drugs), you're more likely to fall asleep at the wheel or have an accident. These herbs may slow cardiac rhythm, lower blood pressure, or make you woozy. And they could aggravate depression, melancholy, and sluggishness. It's always a good idea to slowly introduce a new herb and listen to your body to figure out the right herb, dose, and timing for you. This is especially true for sedatives.

As we've mentioned with other classes of herbs, people's responses may also be highly individualized. My friend can take passionflower to cool her anxiety and rampages by day, but a tiny bit in tea makes *me* need to curl up and take a nap. Some people feel great on hops for sleep while others find their mood darkening if they take it long term.

BEDTIME DOSING TIPS

There are two options for dosing sedative herbs before bedtime: Dose yourself 15 to 30 minutes before you hit the hay, perhaps just before you brush your teeth. Or begin "loading doses" in the evening, taking a low dose of your herb or herbal blend with or after dinner, then again an hour later, and each hour leading up to your bedtime.

Regardless of which option you choose, play around for a few nights to find the doses that work best for you, starting low and building up as needed. You can also keep a bottle of remedies at the bedside to take a half dose if you wake up in the middle of the night and need extra help falling back to sleep.

Tinctures and other liquid extracts are handy and convenient—and they won't add so much fluid that you need to pee in the middle of the night—yet teas and warm milks are comforting and relaxing, perfect for a bedtime ritual. Opt for small yet strongly brewed sleep drinks. Pills work, too, but they're a little slower to break down and take effect and you have less control over the dose.

Also be sure to see the tips for taking herbs in Chapter 6, page 118. For additional safety tips, including for children and for those who are taking medications, pregnant, or lactating, see Chapter 7.

GENTLE SEDATIVES

These first few sedative herbs bridge the relaxant–sedative divide. While you want to be mindful of the aforementioned sedative cautions, these herbs pose less risk than the stronger sedatives that we'll explore later do. The following herbs are an excellent starting point if you'd like deeper relaxation. You can enjoy them as singles, but they also pair well with more gently relaxing and more strongly sedating herbs in formulas.

Chamomile

Matricaria chamomilla
Daisy Family (Asteraceae)

 Well balanced, with effects that are generally helpful day or night. Unlikely to oversedate by day or overstimulate at night.

 Appropriate at night. Unlikely to keep someone awake with stimulating properties; may be more strongly sedating.

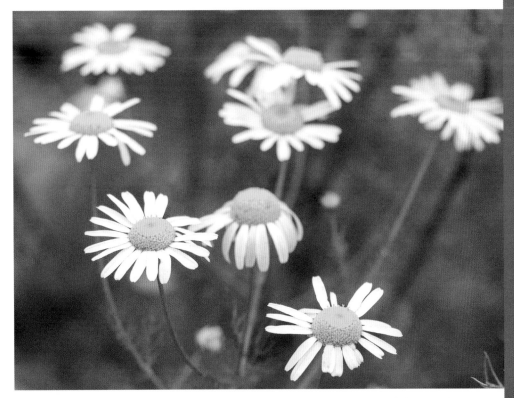

Only the small flower heads are harvested, which means you'll need a lot of plants and time to harvest a sufficient amount. That's why good chamomile can be costly.

Adored Worldwide

You'll find chamomile tea on the shelf in almost every country in the world. It is popular not only in North America and Europe but also throughout Latin America as "manzanilla," in Egypt where most of the world's commercial chamomile is cultivated, and elsewhere. Although many different types of chamomile exist and can be used somewhat interchangeably—including the perennial Roman chamomile (*Chamaemelum nobile*, formerly *Anthemis nobilis*), petal-less pineapple weed (*Matricaria discoidea*), and others across the globe—German chamomile remains the most popular in Western herbal medicine. German chamomile has gone through several Latin name changes, including *Matricaria recutita* and *Chamomilla recutita*.

Sleepy Tea

Chamomile is ubiquitous, safe, and gentle—it's easy to take it for granted or dismiss it. But there's a reason Peter Rabbit's mom served him chamomile tea after a stressful encounter with Farmer McGregor. Several studies confirm chamomile's ability to support sleep quality, allay anxiety, and ease depression, including in elders and in postpartum situations. In one study, chamomile extract was comparable to pharmaceuticals for generalized anxiety disorder. The dose and strength as well as your personal sensitivity will determine whether it simply takes the edge off daytime stress or sends you quickly to bed. Longer, stronger steeps will also increase the bitter and digestive properties. Kids and other people with finicky taste buds will be more amenable to a light steep, which hints of sweet hay, apple, and pineapple and blends well with spearmint or other mints.

Happy Bellies and Fussy Babies

Chamomile is also fantastic where emotional tension brings digestive discomfort and irritability. It is among the most popular herbs for babies and children, highlighting not only the calming but also the bitter digestion-enhancing, carminative, antispasmodic, mildly antimicrobial, and anti-inflammatory actions of this multifaceted flower. Chamomile eases teething pain and irritability, restless sleep, cranky colic, gas, bloating, indigestion, and irritable bowel syndrome; discourages pathogenic gut bacteria; and more. Herbalists often suggest it for "fussy babies of any age." As a flower essence (see page 154), chamomile soothes the solar plexus belly area, quelling anxiety and digestive distress.

Safety and Considerations

Chamomile has a fantastic safety record for all ages; however, some people with daisy-family allergies may react similarly to chamomile. (For those people, catnip offers similar calming and digestive benefits for babies and adults alike.) Small doses as tea appear to be safe in pregnancy.

Working with Chamomile

Chamomile is almost always dried for tea, but it's also lovely in liquid extracts. It makes a superb glycerite or bath "tea" addition. Store-bought tea bags work in a pinch; use several tea bags at once, if needed, to increase the potency. Loose dried chamomile flowers are generally more potent and flavorful than bagged tea, particularly direct from the farm.

Part used: flower head

Tea: 1 heaping teaspoon dried herb/cup, infusion, 1–3 cups daily

    Short steep: pleasant flavor, gentler action

    Long steep: stronger and quite bitter

Tincture or glycerite: 2–5 mL, one to three times daily, solo or in formula

    Fresh 1:2 in 95 percent alcohol or dried 1:5 in 50–60 percent alcohol

Aromatherapy, topical: bath

Recipes: Maria's Sleep Tea (variation), page 123 • Chamomile-Mint Tea, page 127 • Hops Citrus Nightcap Bitters, page 149

Growing and Harvesting Chamomile

This is among the easiest herbs to grow from seed. Direct sow seeds or plugs in well-drained soil in full to part sun, and water moderately throughout the summer. Harvest or deadhead regularly to keep plants producing more flowers; pinch or snip off the flower heads when they're newly open and happy. Get in the mood to enjoy your garden time because it's going to take a while to harvest a decent amount. Use a blueberry rake to speed the process. This is an annual herb, so allow a few flowers to mature and set seed, to self-sow for the next year.

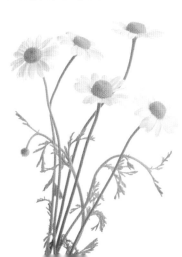

Consider Catnip

The humble catnip (*Nepeta cataria*) offers similar properties to chamomile and is less allergenic, less expensive, and easier to grow and harvest in abundance. The terpene-rich skunky-minty aromas—reminiscent of fellow relaxant herbs valerian, cannabis, hops, lemon balm, and spearmint—and gentle bitterness help calm, ground, and improve digestion. It's more palatable and kid-friendly paired with minty or lemony herbs, sweetened with honey or sugar, or in a sweet base like glycerine. Grow it from seed or plant seedlings. It will likely self-seed and move around your yard year to year, producing ample herbaceous mounds of greenery. Harvest leafy/aerial parts and make medicine as with chamomile. Catnip is perennial in USDA Zones 3–7 and adaptable in dry to slightly moist soil and full sun to partial shade. Harvest and process like lemon balm. Kid- and lactation-friendly, but seek guidance before using when pregnant.

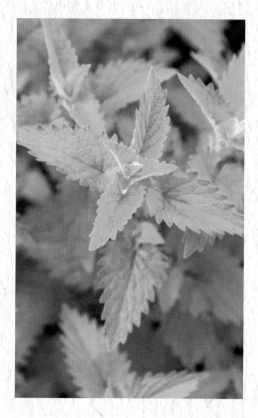

Lavender

Lavandula angustifolia
Mint Family (Lamiaceae)

 Well balanced, with effects that are generally helpful day or night. Unlikely to oversedate by day or overstimulate at night.

 Appropriate at night. Unlikely to keep someone awake with stimulating properties; may be more strongly sedating.

Lavender essential oil has the most research and traditional use—the aroma is inhaled to relieve stress and aid sleep, and the oil is diluted in topical remedies such as lotion or bathwater. It's extremely concentrated and not something easily made at home. It takes approximately 16 pillow-size pounds of lavender buds and fancy distillation equipment to make 1 ounce of essential oil at home—just one drop is equivalent to approximately 30 cups of tea. Less concentrated homemade lavender preparations also work well, and even in this less potent (yet more phytochemically complex) state, lavender is still plenty strong in small doses. You can easily make your own hydrosol, add a pinch of herb to tea blends, craft a tincture, or add the flowers to baths or sleep pillows.

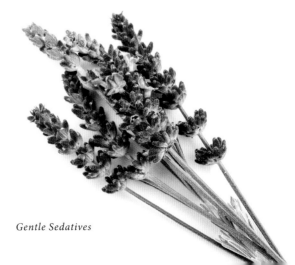

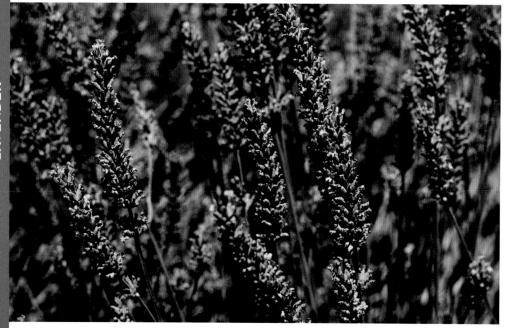

Essential oil remains the easiest and most popular way to work with lavender to promote relaxation and sleep, but you can also make your own remedies with the flower buds.

Mediterranean Nerve Tonic

Lavender's strong aromatics have profound relaxing, energetically moving and dispersive, carminative, pain-relieving, and fast-acting sedative-antidepressant properties whether inhaled, applied topically, or ingested. Consider it for anxiety, sleep, tension headaches, and nervous indigestion, solo or in blends. Although it *may* be nice during the day—especially in tiny doses and in formula—studies find the relaxant properties temporarily hamper cognitive speed. Consider it more at night or for a quick hit of relaxation during a stressful moment,

rather than all day every day. Calming aromatic plants can also help us create our sacred relaxation space or retrain our brain. As a flower essence (see page 154), lavender calms the spirit and the mind—it is one of my favorites for client formulas!

Safety and Considerations

Lavender is a strong plant that doesn't agree with everyone. Don't ingest it while pregnant. The flavor and aroma can be too soapy for some—if you don't enjoy its aroma, consider other relaxing aromatic plants such as holy basil, chamomile, lemon balm, vanilla, or nutmeg instead. Always dilute essential oils—to just 2 percent of the formula or less—before applying topically. I don't recommend using essential oil internally; the flower buds are potent enough and much safer to consume. I'm cautious regarding lavender and essential oils for kids and prefer to limit its use in this population. It may have phytoestrogenic and antiandrogenic actions, disrupting reproductive hormones, and pure essential oils can also be irritating to the skin and hard on the kidneys and liver due to the oils' intense potency.

Working with Lavender

Enjoy fresh or dried. You just need a bit of lavender flowers or remedies—use it as a synergist in blends. Do not consume the essential oil unless it's specially prepared by a reputable company. I prefer remedies made with the crude buds for internal use, because they are more potent and chemically complex.

Part used: buds, flowers

Tea: ½ teaspoon dried herb/cup, infusion, 1–3 cups daily

Tincture: a few drops to 1 mL, one to three times daily, solo or in formula

Fresh 1:2 in 95 percent alcohol or dried 1:5 in 50–60 percent alcohol

Glycerite, syrup, honey, oxymel: ¼–½ teaspoon as needed

Food: add a few buds to sugar, shortbread, chocolate, and in herbes de Provence blends

Aromatherapy: diluted essential oil, hydrosol, bath, inhaled essential oil

Recipes: Maria's Sleep Tea (variation), page 123 • Relief Tincture Blend (variation, flower essence), page 147 • Herbal Sleep Pillow, page 159

Growing and Harvesting Lavender

Lavender is a perennial plant, hardy in USDA Zones 4–9, depending on the species. When planting lavender, seek seedlings and root divisions from varieties known to thrive in your region, then find a sunny, warm spot with somewhat dry, sandy, well-drained soil. Lavender tends to rot out in a standard pampered, watered, mulched garden bed. Cut stems to dry and process to remove the buds, ideally before the buds open. For aromatic remedies, you can include leaves and stems.

California Poppy

Eschscholzia californica
Poppy Family (Papaveraceae)

* *

 Appropriate at night. Unlikely to keep someone awake with stimulating properties; may be more strongly sedating.

Southwestern Indigenous communities have long relied on poppy to induce sleep, mediate pain, and calm agitated nerves. Its safe, nonaddictive constituents produce a mild tranquilizing effect.

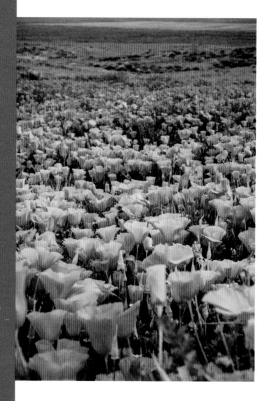

Sleep and Pain

California poppy is helpful for people who wake in the middle of the night and can't go back to sleep, as well as those who struggle with spinning thoughts or pain that interferes with slumber. It gently alleviates many types of pain and can be formulated with other herbs with different constituents for broad-spectrum pain relief. California poppy contains alkaloids that relax, sedate, and ease pain, but does not contain opioids. It's nowhere near as strong as other poppy-family pain relievers such as opium poppy (which is highly addictive and illegal to process for medicine), prickly poppy, and corydalis. As a flower essence (see page 154), California poppy helps ground people in their spiritual awareness

Gentle Sedatives

and connection, reducing their attraction to flashy cultlike mentalities or escapism.

Cough Support

California poppy's relaxing effects also act on the respiratory system, where it can be profoundly effective for coughs, especially coughs that don't respond to the usual cough remedies and those that keep you awake at night. (That said, sometimes it's important to allow a cough to move crud out of the lungs.)

Safety and Considerations

California poppy is one of our safest poppies, kid-friendly and not addictive. It does not appear to show up on drug tests—many herbalists have tested it. Seek the guidance of an herbalist skilled in recovery if you have a history of narcotics addiction. Skip it if you're pregnant or nursing. Use caution when taking it alongside sedating medications.

Working with California Poppy

Best fresh and tinctured (especially in blends), but you can play around with other formats. Preparations that include the root will generally be more potent than those made from just the aerial parts.

Part used: whole plant in flower and seed

Tincture: 1–5 mL, before bed or one to three times daily, solo or in formula

Fresh 1:2 in 95 percent alcohol

Growing and Harvesting California Poppy

As you might assume, a native southwestern US plant that rambles along roadsides in wild fields does not need to be pampered in the garden, but this low-fuss annual prefers a warm, sunny spot without too much competition from other plants. In my chilly, tree-edged yard, it does best in front of the fence and near warm brick paths. Direct sow seeds in late fall (best) or early spring, or plant young plugs—it does not like being moved. Seed packets are readily available from ornamental and medicinal seed companies; skip the fancy cultivars. Mexican gold poppy (*Eschscholzia californica* subsp. *mexicana*) is equivalent. Harvest the whole plant including the translucent orange roots (the strongest part) while it is in flower and seed.

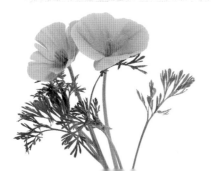

STRONGER SEDATIVE SLEEP AIDS

Although every plant in this book supports sleep, these next herbs are the most famous sleep aids and the most potent sedatives in this book. They're best taken up to 30 minutes before bedtime or via the loading dose method described on page 82. Tinctures act within 15 minutes, while capsules take longer to digest. If you opt for tea, brew it strong and small to prevent nighttime pee breaks. Keep tinctures by the bedside with some water in case you need to redose if you wake too early. Be mindful of all the cautions and other tips mentioned on pages 80–82 for sedatives. These herbs are the most likely to be problematic for some people.

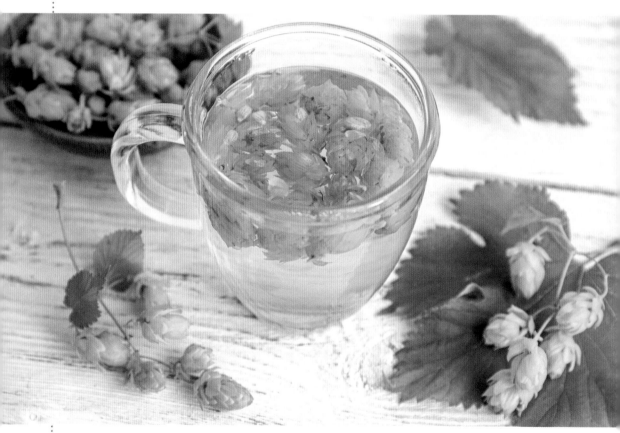

The hop plant's flowerlike strobiles offer profound sedating properties; but they're quite bitter, acidic, and aromatic, like an IPA beer. Very few people enjoy them as tea.

Bedtime Sedating Sleep Support

Passionflower

Passiflora incarnata
Passionflower Family (Passifloraceae)

 Appropriate at night. Unlikely to keep someone awake with stimulating properties; may be more strongly sedating.

This vine rambles throughout the southeastern United States, preferring warm, humid climates. The intricate blooms are mesmerizing. Simply staring into the otherworldly, mandala-like blooms lulls you into tranquil peace and sedation, much like the plant when consumed.

Hypnotic Mandala-Like Flowers

As one of our most reliable, safe sedatives, passionflower brings deep sleep and has become the go-to sedative in my clinical practice, typically in tea or tincture blends. My favorite sleep tea and tincture both feature passionflower; the recipes are on pages 123 and 146. In studies, passion-flower was found to be more effective and broad acting for insomnia compared to other popular sleep herbs, particularly in blends. Several clinical trials have found it to have comparable relaxant effects—with fewer side effects—compared to benzodi-azepine sleep and anxiety medications. It's specific for people who can't shut off their brains due to mind chatter. People prone to anger, frustration, and frenetic energy usually find it a lovely calming, cooling remedy. It can be useful for anxiety solo or in formula, but it may make some people too sleepy, sluggish, or even depressed.

Calming Everywhere

Passionflower gently calms many body systems and can be employed for digestive, cardiac, and respiratory issues related to tension, anxiety, stress, or agitation—for example, stress-induced asthma and hypertension. It is perfect for formulas. As a flower essence (see page 154), pas-sionflower helps you connect to the divine within yourself and follow your creative passions.

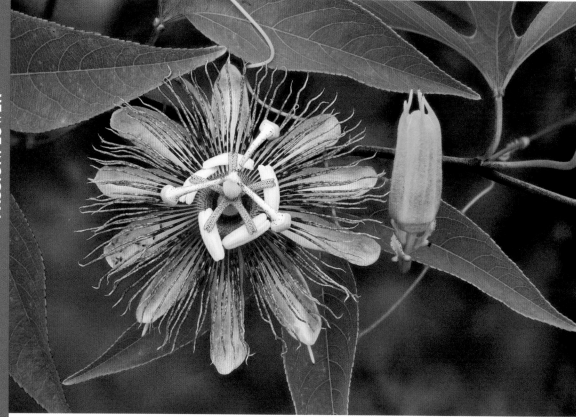

Passionflower's otherworldly blooms, numerology of its flower parts, and heavenly aroma inspired Spanish missionaries in the New World to name this plant after the Passion of Christ.

Safety and Considerations

Ensure you have the *right* passionflower species for sleep; not all species are safe or effective. *Passiflora incarnata* is safe for children, adults, and elders and is one of the most broadly effective sedative herbs for sleep. You'll want to start with low doses to gauge your personal response and ensure it's not *too* sedating (making you groggy, sluggish, depressed, or sleepy during the day). Use caution during pregnancy and when combining with sedative and cardiac drugs.

Working with Passionflower

Use fresh or freshly dried plant material.

Part used: aerial/vine, leaf, flower

Tea: 1 heaping teaspoon dried herb/cup, infusion, 1–3 cups daily or at night

Tincture: 1–5 mL, one to three times daily, solo or in formula

    Fresh 1:2 in 95 percent alcohol (best)

    Dried 1:5 in 50–60 percent alcohol

Syrup, glycerite, oxymel: 1 teaspoon as needed

Capsules/powder: 250–1,000 mg crude herb as needed

Topical: bath

Recipes: Maria's Sleep Tea, page 123 • Maria's Go-To Sleep Tincture Blend, page 146 • Stress Relief Tincture Blend (variation), page 148 • Mellow Me Glycerite, page 152

Growing and Harvesting Passionflower

A perennial in USDA Zones 6–9, passionflower prefers full to part sun and a moderate amount of water. It rambles somewhat aggressively across the southeastern United States, putting forth stunning blooms and edible maypop passionfruit. Many species exist, but only use *P. incarnata* for medicinal use—other species may lack the safety and benefits. It has white petals, a purple/pink fringy crown that is similar in length or longer than the petals, and three-lobed leaves, and the mature fruits turn yellow. Seek the plant from a trustworthy grower. I've seen it labeled incorrectly even by herb growers, but you can trust Strictly Medicinal Seeds for spring-shipped seedlings. Some of my colleagues report that *P. caerulea* is slightly different but still helpful; other species are more typically bred for the fruit or as ornamentals. Grow passionflower in Zones 5 (the northern edge of its range) and 6 by planting it in a protected, warm spot or by bringing it indoors for winter, where it does nicely in a pot, blooming through cold months. In warm climates—like the Southeastern states—this vine can spread out and may become invasive. Cut back aerial parts, preferably while in flower. All aerial parts are medicinal, particularly leaves and flowers.

Valerian

Valeriana officinalis
Honeysuckle Family (Caprifoliaceae)

 Appropriate at night. Unlikely to keep someone awake with stimulating properties; may be more strongly sedating.

In spite of the urban myth, the sedative drug Valium is *not* made from valerian; however, the herb's effects are somewhat similar to the drug's, interacting with GABA receptors to relax us. Valerian is nonaddictive and much safer. Even though valerian is the most studied and most famous herb for sleep, it's also one of the most unreliable across a broad population. Study results are mixed and not particularly impressive—though valerian seems to improve sleep latency (how quickly you fall asleep), and is more effective combined with other sleep herbs. Herbalists take a more nuanced approach and match it to the person's patterns (see "Are You a 'Valerian Person'?," below). I'll share those patterns to guide you, but I also recommend trying valerian in small doses solo first to see how it acts in *your* body.

Are You a "Valerian Person"?

This herb typically suits anxious, thin-framed people who tend to be cold with taut muscles. For "valerian people," it loosens those muscles and supports a deeper, more restorative night's sleep. It was the first herb I tried for sleep when I first came to herbalism, and it worked fantastically. But for others—especially people who are heavier set, run hot, and tend more to anger than worry—it's more likely to make them groggy or agitated and over-stimulated. If that describes you, consider passionflower or hops instead, which have more overtly cooling instead of warming qualities that better balance those "hot people." Passionflower, skullcap, magnolia, lemon balm, and California poppy are

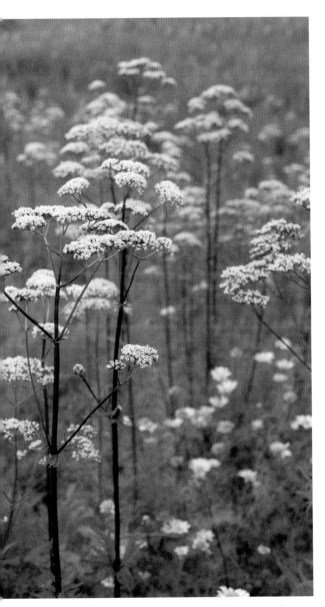

Valerian has sweet-scented flowers and stinky roots that are famous for sleep. It loves to grow in meadows and rampantly self-seeds in fertile soils.

more broadly reliable for most people, in my experience, with passionflower being the strongest. As a flower essence (see page 154), valerian brings deep peace, agreeable and safe whether or not someone is a "valerian type" or on medications.

Muscle-Relaxant Properties

Valerian's muscle-relaxant properties assist pain from tense skeletal muscles, tension headaches, and back pain; they may also ease menstrual cramps and digestive spasm. It offers mild support for reducing blood pressure by relaxing blood vessels. The bigger the dose, the stronger the action. But remember that it will probably also make you sleepy.

Safety and Considerations

All the cautions mentioned on pages 80–82 for sedatives apply to valerian. Slowly introduce the herb, gradually increasing the dose to make sure it agrees with you and doesn't oversedate or agitate. As mentioned above, it's a persnickety plant. While it is kid-friendly, other herbs are more palatable. It's also safe for those who are pregnant or nursing. But I must address its odor. Valerian roots and any remedy made with them *reek* of skunk, body odor, putrefaction, and perfumy dirt. The roots smell worse as they dry, sit out, or are exposed to heat. Some people enjoy the aroma, especially if they associate it

VALERIAN

Stronger Sedative Sleep Aids   97

with a good night's sleep, but most people find it horrendous.

Working with Valerian

Best fresh. You *can* make tea, but it tastes funky and is even more apt to disagree with sensitive people than the tincture is.

Part used: roots

Tincture: 1–5 mL, before bedtime or in formula

Fresh 1:2 in 95 percent alcohol

Glycerite: ¼–1 teaspoon as needed

Growing and Harvesting Valerian

Also called garden heliotrope, valerian grows robustly in the garden (and is, in fact, listed as invasive in some states), with attractive pinkish white blooms, easily reaching 4 to 6 feet tall. It's a perennial in USDA Zones 4–7 and prefers full sun and a moderate amount of water. The sweet honeysuckle-scented blooms contain a hint of the potent skunky aromatics that emanate from the root. This plant self-seeds rampantly and tolerates many soil types, but really takes over in moist manure-rich soil and meadows. Pull up the roots in spring or fall. Usually you can simply grab the whole plant at the base and pull. Spray off dirt, then scrub well with a bristle brush (watch for earthworms). Bigger, older plants have bigger roots. Two-year-old and older plants are preferred, because they're more potent and medicinally complex, but you can also make medicine with the plant babies as you weed them out.

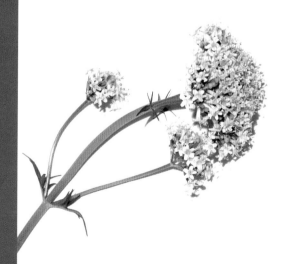

Stronger Sedative Sleep Aids

Hops

Humulus lupulus
Cannabis Family (Cannabaceae)

 Appropriate at night. Unlikely to keep someone awake with stimulating properties; may be more strongly sedating.

The hops plant is among the most potently sedating in our herbal apothecary. It has strongly bitter, aromatic flavors akin to cannabis flowers. Closely related, these dynamic recreational and medicinal herbs have quite a bit in common, particularly the varied and aromatic terpenes that can range from citrus to lavender to pine. Hops lacks the cannabinoids like CBD and THC that make cannabis famous. The flowerlike strobiles hold a powdery yellow substance called lupulin that contains the sedative constituent humulene, alongside other deeply sedating essential oil terpenes including myrcene and caryophyllene.

Cooling Hypnotic and Phytoestrogenic

Remember the poppies scene from the *Wizard of Oz*, when our heroes collapse in a heap of slumber, quickly forgetting the stress and hypervigilance of their mission? That's how I think of hops. The potent, grounding bitter flavor pulls us down into our bodies and then into bed. A cooling herb energetically, it has particular affinity for people who run hot and hot-headed (such as those who don't do well with valerian), and for quelling hot flashes and night sweats that disrupt sleep. Like cannabis, hops is phytoestrogenic, which is particularly helpful for modulating estrogen levels and bolstering dwindling estrogenic activity when someone enters menopause or has their ovaries removed. I often blend hops into the bedtime blends of my perimenopausal clients who are dealing with hot flashes, agitation, insomnia, and other woes of this transition time. It's one of the most popular herbs to add to sleep pillows.

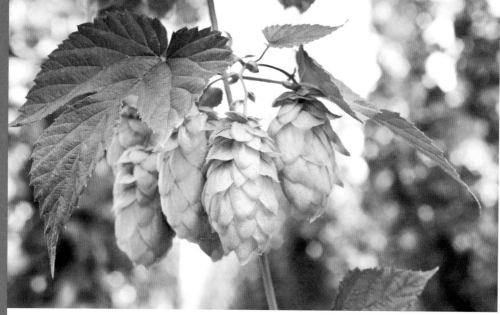

The flowerlike strobiles of this ambling vine not only give IPA beer its characteristically complex citrus-bitter flavors but can also lull you to sleep.

Dynamic Chemistry

Hops is strong, and it does a lot of different things, so it's helpful to be aware of its complex phytochemistry to be sure it's appropriate for you. The intense bitterness boosts digestion and lowers blood sugar. That might be tricky for some people, if they're taking it *right* before bed on an empty stomach, but it would be helpful with dinner, particularly for people dealing with cardiometabolic issues, hunger dysregulation, indigestion, and abdominal weight gain. The phytoestrogenic effects may be great in perimenopause but iffy in men and people who would prefer to affirm masculine hormones. It appears to offer anticancer properties in general but may have proliferative effects on estrogen-sensitive cancers—we don't have quality evidence at this time to clarify. Some people find hops makes them melancholy and depressed with regular use. And although it helps with pain and inflammation, daytime use is often too sedating. We still have a lot to learn about hops medicine, but it's not the right herb for everyone, nor at all times of day.

Safety and Considerations

All the cautions mentioned on pages 80–82 for sedatives apply to hops. Also note the concerns listed above regarding its dynamic chemistry and actions, regarding reproductive hormones, blood sugar, and digestion, that make it less appropriate in certain bodies or at certain times of day.

Working with Hops

Hops medicine is quite bitter and tastes like IPA beer. Fresh plant material is best, but dried is acceptable. Once dried, the strobiles lose potency within a few months. The acidity from alpha and beta acids (which varies by hops variety) will mellow if you store your tincture for a year or more. In recipes, hops blends well with fellow terpene-rich citrus, pine, or lavender.

Part used: ripe strobile

Tea: 1 heaping teaspoon dried strobiles/cup, infusion, 4–8 ounces at night (if you tolerate the flavor)

Tincture: 1–5 mL, before dinner or at bedtime

Fresh 1:2 in 95 percent alcohol (best) or freshly dried 1:5 in 70–75 percent alcohol (High-proof alcohol best extracts the constituents; I rough-chop the strobiles in a blender or food processor with the alcohol.)

Syrup, glycerite, oxymel: 1 teaspoon as needed

Capsules/powder: 250–1,000 mg crude herb as needed

Recipes: Hops Citrus Nightcap Bitters, page 149 • Lazy Bitters (variation), page 149 • Herbal Sleep Pillow, page 159

Growing and Harvesting Hops

This perennial vine is hardy in USDA Zones 5–9; it prefers full sun and doesn't require a lot of water. It grows vigorously each season, gripping and swirling up fence lines and strings, so give it plenty of room to grow, checking on it periodically to retwirl it in the directions you want it to climb. One of my beer-making friends directed it over his patio to provide shade in summer. Hops is easy to grow from cuttings. Because of the beer industry, many cultivars exist; all have medicinal benefit and support sleep but will vary widely in aroma, bitterness, and acid content (the acidity mellows as it ages). If you want more strongly sedating hops, seek "bittering" varieties (used for bittering beer) with higher amounts of the terpenes mentioned above. You can cut it back after harvesting—it will regrow in spring. Whole books have been written about selecting and growing hops for homebrewing. Harvest the flowerlike strobile cones, which are the mature fruiting body, in late summer or autumn once mature. You'll know they're ready when they snap like a carrot when broken and you see lots of powdery yellow lupulin inside. It's best fresh, though it will keep for a few months if carefully dried.

Additional Sleep Remedies

Beyond herbs, these other home remedies and dietary supplements are also worthy of merit.

MELATONIN

A popular sleep aid on its own and in sleep blends, supplemental melatonin may boost your natural production of this sleep hormone. While generally safe, it doesn't agree with or work for everyone. It's most effective to help you fall asleep and the effects can wear off quickly. It may also help us reset after jet lag, help older kids who are on the autism spectrum with sleep-cycle difficulties, support immune resistance to infections and cancer, decrease inflammation, uplift and calm mood, and improve estrogen production in perimenopausal people. It may also enhance sphincter tone in acid reflux and reduce age-related bladder tone and urination symptoms—but the evidence for this is still preliminary and mixed. A sustained-release supplement, taken a few hours before bedtime, will better mimic your body's natural release of melatonin. A typical adult dose ranges from 1 to 5 mg, starting on the low end. Evidence suggests that you will not build a tolerance to it. Melatonin may cause more vivid (potentially nightmarish) dreams for some people because it increases REM sleep time. Higher doses are more likely to cause daytime drowsiness, especially among elders. Do not use melatonin in young children; it may also be inappropriate for elders with dementia and in untreated sleep apnea.

TART CHERRY JUICE

Cherries are among the few foods that contain small quantities of melatonin, and studies suggest that drinking a serving of tart cherry juice in the morning and evening supports your own melatonin levels and overall sleep quality. Tart cherry juice also has gout-relieving and -preventive properties and anti-inflammatory properties, particularly for postexercise exertion. It's best with long-term daily consumption. The studies used 8-ounce servings of juice, but I prefer 1 ounce of the organic concentrate—this is equivalent to 8 ounces of juice, it's more convenient, and it's easy to mix into recipes such as Tart Cherry Soda (page 129) or add as a purposeful sweetener to smoothies and chia pudding. Be mindful of the sugar content, which may not agree with everyone.

Bedtime Sedating Sleep Support

TRYPTOPHAN, 5-HTP, OR ST. JOHN'S WORT

These serotonin boosters may enhance mood, ease anxiety, and support sleep when taken in the morning and/or daytime. Not everyone responds well to a serotonin boost, and these can interact with numerous serotonin-boosting medications. St. John's wort has many additional herb–drug interactions, often clearing drugs out of the system too quickly, as well as nuances as a nervine (see page 76 for more). I don't tend to turn to these supplements for sleep support specifically, but some people find them helpful, and you'll often find one or more in dietary supplement sleep and relaxation blends.

MAGNESIUM

This important mineral has hundreds of functions throughout the human body, and most of us consume suboptimal amounts in our diets. Deficiency can lead to tense or spastic muscles and nerve issues, and many people find that they sleep more deeply if they boost their magnesium intake at night. Favorite forms include magnesium citrate, magnesium glycinate, or chelated magnesium. If you take too much, it will give you loose stools—back down the dose if that happens. Herbalist and nutritionist Paul Bergner also recommends an effective

and inexpensive (but *terrible*-tasting) combination of 1 ounce plain milk of magnesia mixed with about 4 ounces of apple cider vinegar. Stir the mixture; if it's not clear after 5 minutes, add a little more vinegar until it turns clear. A chemical reaction will occur, and the final liquid contains approximately 40 mg of easily absorbed magnesium and can be taken in tablespoon doses added to water.

Herbal and food sources of magnesium include oat straw, nettle leaf, oat bran, almonds, cashews, cacao nibs, and dark leafy greens—though these foods typically contain less than 100 mg of magnesium per serving.

L-THEANINE

Theanine is an amino acid extracted from green tea, which is one reason why green tea tends to cause less jitteriness than coffee does, even though it contains a small amount of caffeine. Theanine extracts are caffeine-free and tend to have a gentle yet therapeutic relaxant effect that is generally well tolerated day or night. It's often found in relaxing supplement blends, functional foods, even sleepy-time cannabis gummies. As a solo dietary supplement, theanine is relatively inexpensive and well tolerated by most. A typical starting dose is 100 mg.

WARM HONEY MILK

This old home remedy is quite soothing and tasty before bed or if you're having a restless night. It may work by mildly boosting tryptophan. Be mindful of the sugar effect if you tend toward blood sugar roller coasters that disrupt sleep. See my recipe on page 139.

WHAT ABOUT CANNABIS?

As the regulatory and cultural landscape shifts, interest in both THC- and CBD-dominant cannabis strains for medicine has boomed. Stress, anxiety, sleep, pain, inflammation, and migraines are among the most popular reasons why people turn to cannabis for medicine. Many of my clients and colleagues—particularly those who live in states where it's completely legal—report that cannabis has done wonders for their sleep, sometimes helping them to wean off various medications (with their doctor's supervision). The topic of medicinal cannabis is too vast for me to cover in this book. I highly recommend herbalist Tammi Sweet's books and online courses (see Resources, page 178). But here are a few tips if you're interested in working with cannabis for sleep.

Combining THC, CBD, and Other Herbs
High-CBD/low-THC "hemp flower" cannabis is legal in most states. Its effects are more subtle.

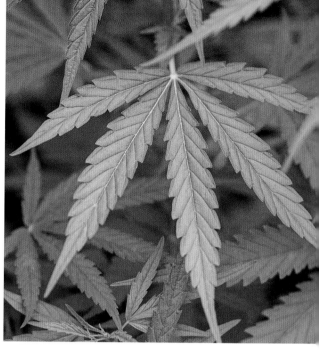

Studies and anecdotal reports suggest that cannabis remedies may support sleep and ease anxiety.

THC-dominant cannabis strains have more profound euphoric and relaxant "high" effects. For sleep and anxiety, you often benefit by using a much lower dose than what most people use recreationally. Seek strains that are more relaxing if your goal is sleep, and remember that everyone responds a little differently.

A 1:1 combination of THC and CBD—which can be made with isolates or by combining THC- and CBD-dominant strains together—may produce more even-keeled and therapeutic support with less of a high. Specialty products may include sedating constituents CBN, myrcene, linalool, caryophyllene, and terpinolene, or other calming herbs and remedies.

Seek products made with whole-plant constituents or that market the "entourage" effect—these will often achieve better results at lower doses by combining multiple cannabinoids and terpenes versus a high dose of one lab-isolated THC or CBD cannabinoid.

Cannabis blends well with other medicinal herbs, such as the ones we've discussed in this book. Some companies combine them in formula for purchase, too. You may be able to get better calming effects by combining a smaller dose of cannabis along with other relaxing herbs.

Tips for Use
Inhaled cannabis will take effect almost immediately but will also taper off more quickly. Edibles and tinctures typically take between 45 minutes and 150 minutes to kick in but the effects will linger longer in the body.

* If cannabis makes you snack incessantly, consider taking it *just* before you go to bed, which can also limit the blood sugar roller coaster of those snacks that may disrupt sleep.

* Give yourself plenty of time on a weekend to test and find your dose on a new batch, taking just a tiny amount (a few drops), waiting several hours, taking a few more if needed, waiting several more hours, and so on. The best dose is the minimum dose that gives you the desired benefits. Taking higher doses poses a greater risk for side effects, habituation, and withdrawal, and may simply be unnecessary.

* Be careful combining cannabis with medications or alcohol. I know several people who fainted from syncope by unintentionally taking relatively large amounts of THC cannabis alongside a glass or two of alcohol. The episode is generally temporary and harmless (unless you injure yourself during the fall) but not ideal. Cannabis—particularly high-THC forms—may also worsen sleep apnea and disrupt daytime function.

Make Your Own Remedies
Tammi Sweet's books and courses will teach you how to grow and make your own cannabis remedies. The processes are very similar to those in this book, except that you'll usually want to decarboxylate the dried flowers before making medicine with them. To decarboxylate (which converts the cannabinoids into CBD and THC), dry roast them in a closed container at 250°F (121°C) for 80 minutes, stirring frequently, or a slightly lower temperature for longer. High-proof alcohol or olive or coconut oil are the best solvents for decarbed cannabis, but you can also make tea or gummies, extract in glycerine, or cook into baked goods.

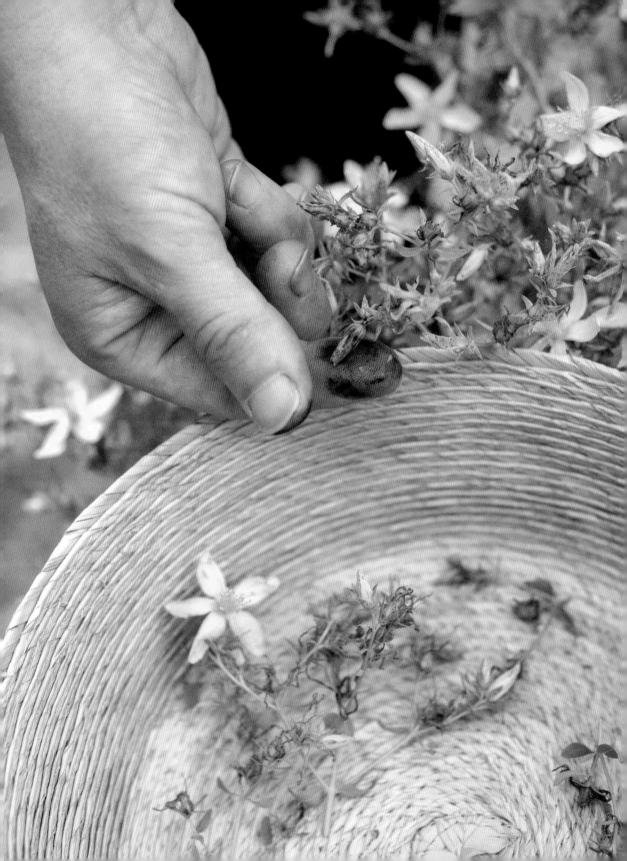

CHAPTER 5

Harvesting and Drying Herbs

Growing (or, in some cases, wildcrafting) and harvesting your own herbs will provide you with the most exceptional herbal medicine quality anywhere *and* a deep, healing connection with the plants directly. However, it's not essential to grow your own herbs to make your own herbal remedies—you can purchase dried and fresh herbs direct from herb farms or seek ingredients on the bulk loose herb market. In this chapter we'll explore some basic harvesting techniques, and you can refer to the growing tips in individual plant profiles in this book. For more growing information, refer to Resources on page 178.

In a pinch or just starting out? Many wonderful companies sell premade products and blends. That's how I started out. See page 178 for tips on sourcing herbs and my favorite farms, companies, and brands.

Harvesting Herbs

If you're growing or wildcrafting your own herbs, you'll need to harvest them at the right time for maximum potency. Generally speaking, harvest when the plant looks, smells, and tastes potent, flavorful, healthy, and vital—basically, when it's "happy." Aromatic herbs possess more flavor when they're harvested earlier in the day. If you're planning to dry herbs, harvest them after the dew has evaporated (and, if you're relying on warm, sunny weather for the dehydration process, check the forecast). Harvest flowers just as they open. Harvest roots and barks in spring or fall. That's the *ideal* scenario, but fit this process into your schedule. If that means you're out there late at night with a headlamp jumping at a frost warning or digging a root in mid-June, so be it!

LEAVES AND AERIAL PARTS

Aerial refers to the aboveground parts of the plant, which may be in flower or not. Harvest in a way that encourages future growth while also giving you enough material for making remedies.

For herbs with leaves and stems that branch off from the main stem (most

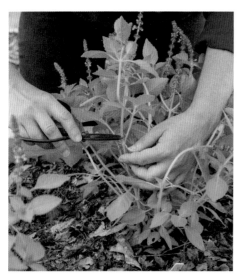

Pinching off branching herbs (like this holy basil) just above a leaf node will encourage future, bushier growth. Be sure to leave a few sets of leaves behind.

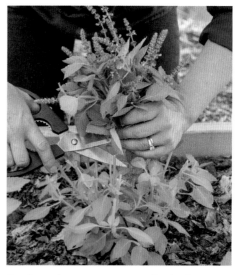

For faster harvests, you can give herbs a "bad haircut" by hacking across the top one-third to two-thirds of the herb.

Harvesting and Drying Herbs

plants), harvest the top one-third to two-thirds of the plant, making sure to leave at least a few sets of leaves behind. The plant will look and recoup better if you trim *just* above a leaf node—this is where the new growth will take place. That said, if you're short on time, have a lot of plant material to harvest, or are working with a sprawling plant like thyme, you can give it a "bad haircut": Bunch the material together in your hands, and hack across the top portion in a straight line. The plant will look scraggly at first but grow back just fine.

For plants that do not branch or leaf out—such as oat straw, chives, parsley, and lemongrass stalks—you'll instead cut stems right down to the ground, but leave one-third to two-thirds of the plant untouched. Chives, oat straw, and lemongrass's grassy tops (not the tightly rolled stalk part) can also be trimmed from the top.

FLOWERS AND BUDS

Pinch off the newly opened blossoms, including any green sepals or bracts at the base of the flower. Typically, the whole flower head is left intact (chamomile), but you may opt to remove only the petals (rose). When drying flowers, lay them out in a single layer and consider using a dehydrator. You want to make sure the

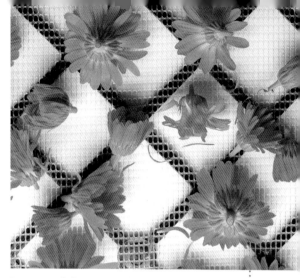

Leaves and flowers are best dried between 95 and 110°F (35 and 43°C). Arrange flowers in a single layer in the dehydrator to ensure the middles dry thoroughly.

middles are completely dried or they will ferment and mold in storage.

BARK

Harvest bark in early spring when the sap is rising but the tree hasn't yet leafed out, or in fall once the leaves have begun to change color and drop. In a pinch, though, you *could* harvest bark at any time of the year—for example, when you're pruning the tree for vigor and shape. The medicinal part of bark is the inner bark, not the outer bark (which is more astringent and protective for the plant) nor the inner woody pith. The inner bark is often juicy, green, and aromatic.

Do not remove bark directly from a live tree. Prune the branches off first, aiming for twigs and branches up to approximately 1½ inches in diameter—you won't need to remove the outer bark from these young branches. How you prune will determine the tree or shrub's future growth. A "heading cut" is made above a strong node and will encourage the tree to bush out from that spot. A "thinning cut" removes the branch to the base of the trunk, junction, or the

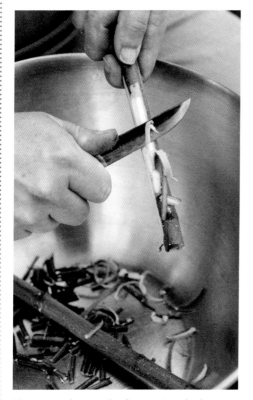

The greenish inner bark contains the best medicine. Young branches can be stripped of bark without having to worry about removing the darker outer bark.

ground. You may opt to take down a whole tree or take advantage of a blow-down after a storm; you'll need to remove the outer bark from wider branches and the trunk. I prefer harvesting bark from smaller branches and twigs—it's easier.

If there are any leaves on the pruned limbs, pull those off. Then use a knife or peeler to scrape off the bark and use clippers to trim up the twigs—this is what you'll use to make medicine. Sometimes the bark peels off easily, and you can just slice it down the length or mash it a bit between two rocks, then strip it by hand.

If you decide to tincture bark, consider adding 10 percent glycerine (or honey) during maceration or after pressing. Bark is usually rich in astringent tannins, which bind to other constituents and precipitate out, making your tincture gloppy and less potent over time. Glycerine helps stabilize and stall the process.

ROOTS

As with bark, roots are best dug up in spring or fall rather than when the plant is focused on putting out leafy growth and flowers, yet exceptions can be made if needed.

A garden fork loosens the soil around the plant and may suffice for digging up the roots. Depending on the plant and land, use a sharp spade or hori hori knife, particularly good for slicing a chunk off

Harvesting and Drying Herbs

of a root crown. For lighter travel and finer details (but more effort on your part) you can work out the root with a digging stick, hori hori, or CobraHead weeder. These do well for roots that travel, like burdock and nettle, or those that are not hard to bring up, like mullein and valerian.

Once you've got your roots out of the ground, bang them against the ground or a rock to loosen and remove some dirt. Rinse them off with the powerwash setting of your garden hose sprayer and/or dunk them in cold water and swish them around vigorously. If dirt remains, remove it with a potato scrubber and cold water. Roots should be processed fresh. Chop roots into smaller pieces with a hatchet, loppers, clippers, or wood chipper to dehydrate them or use fresh.

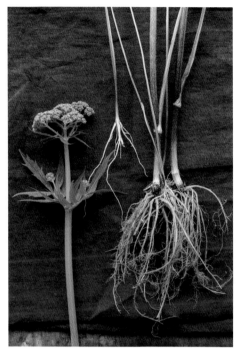

The roots of valerian are most often consumed for sleep, though the flower essence is also of value.

Should I Wash My Herbs?

Except for roots, we usually *don't* wash herbs. That's because introducing water will increase the risk of spoilage for drying herbs and several types of herbal preparations (glycerites, honeys). Simply ensure you're picking plants that are relatively clean (from dirt, pollen, animal manure, pollutants) and discard any questionable material.

If your plants are dirty, wash them off with a hose *before* you harvest them, let them air-dry, then harvest them. If you've harvested herbs that really do need to be cleaned, use cold water and a salad spinner, gently towel dry, then let them finish air-drying before proceeding with your processing. If you can dust off the dirt with a clean, dry brush or towel, do that instead. Roots should be washed in cold water.

Drying Herbs

Keep dried herbs on hand for making tea, cooking, and year-round remedy making. It's cheap and easy to dry herbs, particularly if you're not sure when or how you want to use them later. Most dried herbs, flowers, and fruits keep for a least 1 year in good storage conditions (see page 115), and longer for roots, bark, and mushrooms. Dried herbs often keep even longer; most of what you buy online and in stores is already 1 to 3 years old. As long as your dried herbs still look, smell, and taste good, you can use them.

Dried herbs can take up a considerable amount of pantry and cabinet space, though. *Most* herbs can be used fresh or dried, with a few that are best fresh or best dried.

Herbs best used fresh or freshly dried. Milky oat seed, St. John's wort, and motherwort are vastly superior when used fresh. Dried skullcap, lemon balm, California poppy, and valerian can be used in recipes but will not be anywhere near as strong or effective as their fresh counterparts. Passionflower and linden make lovely dried herbs but lose potency more quickly than other dried herbs (in 3 to 8 months). Take extra-special care when drying these herbs to maintain maximum quality. In general, make tinctures with fresh plants if you have the option, dried if you don't.

Dried versus Fresh

There's a time and place for both. Here are some general guidelines for formulations:

DRIED HERBS	FRESH HERBS
Tea	Aromatic teas in summer
Spice cabinet/seasoning mixes	Infused water, seltzer
Oxymels*	Tinctures
Glycerites*	Cooked honeys
Tinctures	Cooking
Honey (especially raw)*	
Vinegars*	

*You can use either fresh or dried herbs for these products, but bear in mind that introducing moisture from fresh plants will increase the risk of spoilage. Wilting the fresh herb for a few hours before making a "best dry" recipe limits the spoilage risk.

Harvesting and Drying Herbs

DRYING METHODS

Every herbalist will offer a different "best" way to dry herbs. The best method for *you* will depend on convenience, materials, space, climate, and the plant (and part) you're drying. Flowers, roots, and berries should be dried in a single layer. Leave aerial parts on the stem, use flowers whole, and chop the roots. (Some roots are impossible to chop once dried.)

Your goal: thoroughly crisp-dry plants that easily crumble, pull off from the stem, or break into pieces. Any residual moisture could ferment or rot the plant in storage; this is a particular problem for flower heads and berries. If you're unsure, put a few in a jar or plastic bag and place in the sun to see if moisture collects—if so, it's not dry enough. Once your plant is dried, remove it promptly to process and store. Herbs get dusty and less potent if they sit around too long. Your primary drying methods include the following.

Air-Drying

In the iconic herbal kitchen, herbs hang by the rafters or over the woodstove, drying in bundles. Bring a few stems together with string or an elastic band to hang them from pegs, or lay them flat on screens, preferably in a well-ventilated, dry area, out of direct sunlight. Fans and collapsible herb drying racks are handy for this. Air-drying works best for leaves

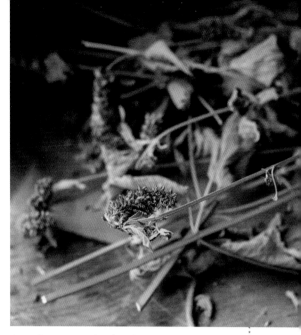

Aerial parts can be dried or crisped in a paper bag in a warm car to improvise a dehydrator environment.

and flowers and (if the air is dry enough) chopped roots, though they could take a few days to a week or longer. Use it for juicy herbs like basil that turn black easily during the drying process. Air-drying works well if your air is dry. In high humidity, tough herbs won't get crisp-dry at room temperature. You could start your plants with air-drying to remove most of the moisture, then use a low-heat method to crisp them.

Low-Heat Drying

As humidity increases, bump up the heat and ventilation to dry your plants. Ideal maximum drying temperature for most herbs runs from 95 to 110°F (35 to 43°C) depending on the plant and ambient humidity (higher for fruit and roots). Low-heat methods dry herbs quickly, which may actually result in better-quality dried herbs versus those left to sit for days or weeks air-drying. Check your plants every 6 to 24 hours and move them around if some areas are drying faster than others. Commercial herb growers construct drying sheds, hoop houses covered with shade cloth, or tobacco trailers to dry herbs this way. Once dry, the herbs should be immediately removed, processed, and stored.

Here are some other low-budget techniques for the backyard herbalist.

Paper Bag in the Car

This is my favorite method for aerial parts and leaves! (That said, with our increasing heat and humidity, I now start with air-drying and then move them to the "car dehydrator" for a final crisping.) Loosely pack your bag with herbs, cinch it shut with a clothespin, and place it in the windshield of your car on a warm, sunny day. (If it's hot out, place the bags on the car seat or in a clean trunk.) Crack the window if it's really hot or your plants are particularly juicy. The bag protects the plant from direct sunlight and helps wick away moisture. A basket of herbs with another basket over it also works. Remove, process, and store promptly once dried.

Dehydrator

Make sure your dehydrator is good quality and able to hit 95 to 110°F (35 to 43°C) for leaves and flowers, 125 to 135°F (52 to 57°C) for fruit, and somewhere in between for roots and mushrooms. Cheap dehydrators tend to get too hot, which is a particular problem for aromatic plants. If you notice a strong herb smell, it's too hot. Always get a bigger dehydrator than you think you'll need! Dry herbs in a single layer. Roots, fruit, and flowers dry *best* in a dehydrator. For herbs like basil and comfrey that turn black easily, make sure the dehydrator is not too hot and your plants are in a single layer. The Excalibur brand is good but pricey. Resourceful people make their own. Make sure you can control the temperature. Remove, process, and store promptly once dried.

Other Methods

Some people use the oven and the microwave, but these are too hot for most herbs. Attics, sheds, and greenhouses work well. Hang herbs from a clothesline or suspended screens/racks or in brown paper bags. Make sure your drying space is clean, won't rust, and is free of pests like mice and rats, and that you don't forget about your herbs. Any method that involves heat (even low heat, like the car) will require attentiveness to promptly remove, process, and store once dried—letting them linger in the heat will reduce potency.

GARBLING DRIED HERBS

"Garbling" is the technical term (yes, really) for processing dried herbs to remove the leaves from the stem and break everything up into small "cut and sifted" pieces. The less broken down a plant is, the better it retains its quality in storage, but it's far easier to use your herbs if they're broken down a bit, and you can fit more material in a jar once they're cut and sifted.

Once your herbs are crisp-dry, hold them over a large bowl or bin and garble by hand, stripping the leaves off the stem and removing any additional large stems (for prickly nettle or motherwort, wear clean gloves). Then crumble the herbs with your hands.

Or create a "rubbing screen": Cover a box or bin with galvanized hardware cloth, stainless steel mesh, or a plastic screen (something that won't rust) and rub the herbs back and forth so that the broken leaves fall through into the bin while the stems remain on top for easy removal. You may want different sizes of mesh for different plants.

Store flowers, fruits, roots, and mushrooms exactly as they come out of the dehydrator—no garbling necessary. You

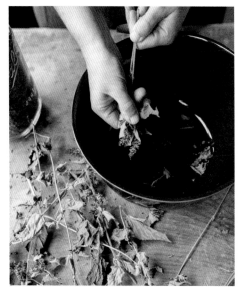

Once your herb is totally crisp-dry, "garble" the herb by removing the leaves and flowers from the stems.

may be able to more finely chop roots and mushrooms with a bullet-style grinder, wood chipper, blender, or meat grinder.

STORING DRIED HERBS

Heat, light, oxygen, and moisture degrade the quality of your herbs. Store dried herbs and shelf-stable remedies in a cool, dark, dry spot like a pantry or cabinet. Glass jars with tight-fitting lids work best. If you don't plan to use an herb for several months, use a mason jar vacuum sealer to further enhance the shelf life. This option isn't practical if you plan to open the jar more often.

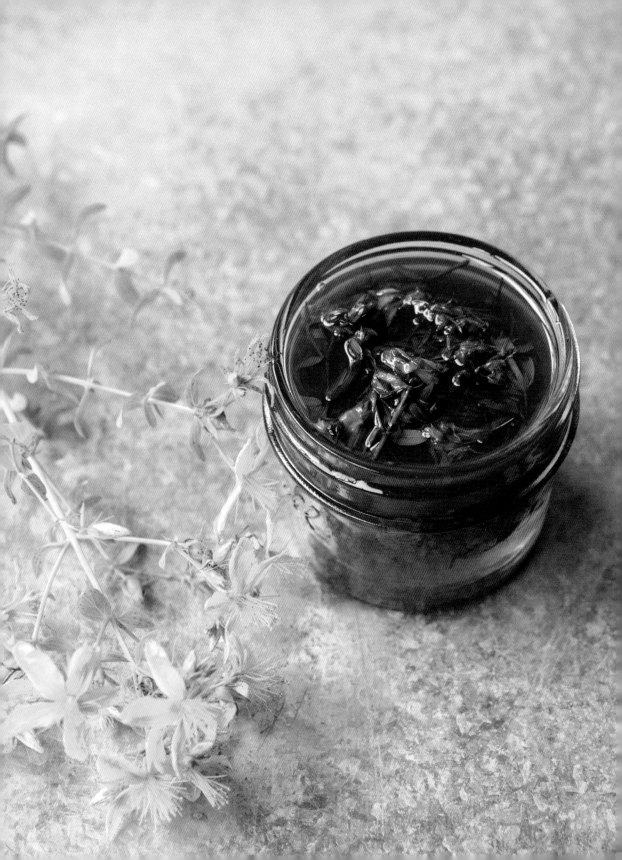

CHAPTER 6

Sleep-Support Recipes and Remedies

Craft stellar herbal remedies in your kitchen that surpass anything you can buy in stores. It's amazingly easy and fun. The basic method for most recipes: Shove herbs in a jar, cover them with something (e.g., alcohol, vinegar, honey), then strain them after a few weeks. Or simmer them on the stove, then strain them. As my teacher Michael Moore would say, "This isn't rocket science, it's herbology!"

Tips for Taking Herbs

Here are some very basic guidelines for using herbs as medicine. When in doubt, please don't hesitate to seek professional guidance, especially if your condition is serious or worsens.

CHOOSING HERBS, FORMULAS, AND RECIPES

Sometimes it can be tricky to figure out which herbs and formulas in the sea of options will be right for *you*. I'm hoping that the plant profiles and general information in the preceding chapters will help you learn about each plant so that you can better understand their actions and nuances, and that you'll have narrowed them down to one or a few that sound like the best options for *you* as an individual.

You can certainly opt to work with "simple" herbs—that is, just one *single* herb in a tea, tincture, pill, or other format. You might find your perfect herbal ally, and working with single herbs allows you to better understand how that plant affects you.

But formulas are also fun and may enhance or balance herbs in a way that improves their flavor or efficacy. By better understanding your sleep-support herbs through our prior chapters, you'll be able to assess commercial formulas to pick one that feels best targeted to *your* needs, or pick one or two of my own favorite recipes from the pages to come to begin crafting your own formulas. It's probably a good idea to start with just one or two herbal remedies, whether single herbs or formulas. Feel free to tinker and make the recipes your own!

You'll hopefully notice some improvement within just a few days, with deeper effects over time, unless it's one of the slower-acting herbs like milky oat, bacopa, St. John's wort, or gotu kola, that usually take a few months to kick in. If an herb or formula doesn't agree with you, that will typically be apparent within a few days. And if it's been two or three months and you're really not seeing any difference, it's time to switch things up and/or seek professional guidance.

START LOW AND SLOW

When starting out with a new herb or recipe, make or buy small batches until you know what works best for you. Take your first dose on a weekend and start with a very low dose—such as just a few drops of tincture, a pinch of tea, or a quarter cup of tea—then gradually increase your dose over the coming days to determine how your body responds to the herb and which dose feels best. If it's a more energizing herb, begin by taking it only in the morning. If it's a more calming or sedating herb, first try it in the evening. Listen to your body. It will tell you which herbs and doses are right for you.

The exact dose that you need of an herb will vary depending on the person, the herb, the preparation, and even the practitioner. Sometimes just a few drops of a well-chosen herb will elicit a favorable response, and many herbalists prefer these almost-homeopathic doses. On the other side of the spectrum, TCM herbalists often prefer to hit things heavy with large doses of herbs. Don't let this get overwhelming; herbs work well in a wide range of doses.

LISTEN TO YOUR BODY

Pay attention to how you *feel* when you take a remedy. At first you might just get a vague sense that it resonates with you—or it doesn't. As time goes on, are you getting the desired effects? Any other changes?

If you notice a negative side effect, stop taking the remedy. Do your research: Is this reaction common or known? Depending on the reaction, consider trying the remedy again once or twice more to confirm whether it was caused by the remedy. If you do have a negative side effect from the herb, stop taking it or seek professional guidance. Take note and

be cautious with herbs that have similar actions or are related.

If you're not seeing results from the recommended dose within a reasonable amount of time (this varies by herb and condition, but some improvements will generally be seen within 1 to 2 weeks), consider increasing the dose. If you're not seeing results within a month or two, consider different herbs or therapies.

Most herbs do best taken with food, especially if you have a sensitive stomach. This is particularly true for bitter, strong-tasting, or astringent herbs, as well as those that lower blood sugar (hypoglycemic herbs).

If you notice that you're not sleeping well while taking a remedy, consider taking it earlier in the day or find a different herb or formula. For the herbs mentioned in this book, some people may find ashwagandha or reishi too stimulating at night or too stimulating at any time of day, while many others find them helpful. In sleep apnea or some sleep disorders, the more sedating and relaxant herbs may aggravate these conditions and worsen sleep.

For additional safety tips, including for children and for those who are taking medications, pregnant, or lactating, see Chapter 7.

Herbal Beverages

Water-based beverages allow you to easily incorporate herbs into your daily life. For these recipes I've chosen to focus on my favorite flavor profiles and have avoided those like hops and valerian that may have efficacy but taste gross. The simple act of making and sipping these recipes should bring joy and pleasure, which will only enhance the stress-relieving, sanctuary-creating benefits of the herbs. If you're drinking an herbal beverage before bedtime, stick to smaller, stronger doses so you aren't waking up in the middle of the night to pee. You can also add herbal extracts like tinctures, vinegar, honey, glycerite, or oxymel to your beverages. But let's start with my favorite ways to infuse herbs directly in water.

Aside from eating plants directly, extracting them in water is the purest, simplest, most affordable, easiest way to take medicinal herbs. Hot water extracts a wide range of constituents from a plant, including aromatics and minerals, delivering them in an easily digested form. Most of our herbal remedies involve extracting constituents with a solvent. In the case of water, it's hydrating, healthy, gentle, and safe for anyone.

TEA-FRIENDLY HERBS

Many of our relaxing sleep herbs smell or taste unpleasant, making them less suitable for tea. Here are some of the most tea-friendly sippers from this book that either taste good or are easy enough to spruce up with flavorful herbs.

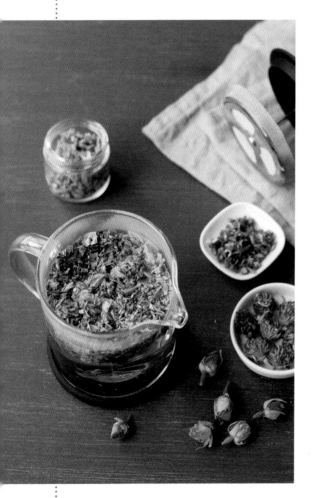

Sleep-Support Recipes and Remedies

- Holy basil (yum!)
- Lemon balm
- Linden (yum!)
- Lavender (just a little!)
- Skullcap (slightly bitter)
- Passionflower
- Chamomile (bitter with long steeps)
- Catnip (a bit bitter)
- Oat straw or tops
- Mimosa
- Ashwagandha
- Reishi (bitter)
- Rose (yum! sprinkle in)
- Vanilla (yum!)
- Nutmeg (yum! just a pinch!)

Iced Tea, Two Ways

Why not try your herbal tea iced? It tastes great in summertime and hot climates. Here are a couple of ways to make it. Add extra panache to your iced tea by freezing your favorite teas in ice cube trays to add to iced tea or purée into frozen drinks and smoothies. For garnish, you can freeze sprigs of herbs or flowers—such as chamomile, lavender, rosemary, and lemon balm—into ice cube trays.

Double strength. Brew your tea as you would for a hot tea (see page 122 for infusion and page 131 for decoction), but use twice the plant material. Strain your tea over ice cubes. Make sure to do this in a container that can handle heat and cold simultaneously—most ceramic and glass vessels will break, but tempered glass and stainless steel should hold up.

Chill it. If you've got time to plan ahead, brew your tea as you normally would, then transfer the strained tea to the fridge until it's cold. Serve over ice.

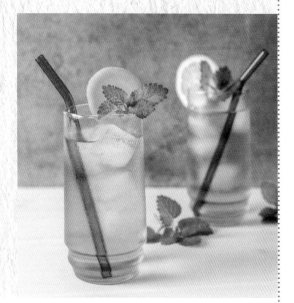

Making a Tea Infusion

When we infuse herbs, we *steep* them in water, typically hot water. Leaves, flowers, and aromatic plants—those that are delicate and offer their medicine easily—should be steeped. They may lose potency with simmering. Dried herbs usually lend themselves better to the water extraction than fresh plants do. French press pots, in-mug infusers, and teapots or travel mugs with stainless strainers for infusion work well for this. Feel free to play around with how much herb you use, how hot the water is, and how long it steeps—it all works, but you'll notice subtle differences in strength and flavor.

1 heaping teaspoon to 1 heaping tablespoon dried herb

Suggested tools: vessel, strainer/infuser, mug

1. Place your herb in the vessel, cover with 8–16 ounces of near-boiling water. If desired, cover the vessel as it steeps (which will hold the aromatics in, though this isn't absolutely necessary).

2. Strain and drink. The duration of steeping will depend on the plant. Unlike true tea, most herbs should be steeped for at least 10 to 15 minutes and will tolerate much longer steeping times (even hours). If you're including high-mucilage (such as marshmallow) or mineral-rich (such as nettle or oat straw) herbs in the blend, steeping them for 4 to 12 hours will better extract those constituents.

3. Refrigerate any extras for up to 2 to 3 days.

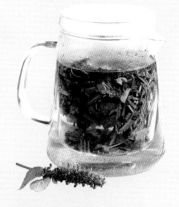

VARIATIONS

Fresh herb infusion: While most herbs infuse best dry, aromatic herbs like holy basil and lemon balm work well fresh, but you'll need more plant material and time. Unless you want a really light infusion, use a handful of herb per 16 ounces of water and infuse for 20 minutes. Refrigerate extras for 1 to 2 days.

Cold water infusion/seltzer: This makes a very light, refreshing, hydrating beverage that highlights the plant's flavorful aromatics. Steep approximately 3 large sprigs of fresh herb per liter of water or plain seltzer for 30 minutes. Refrigerate extras, and drink within 6 to 12 hours.

Maria's Sleep Tea

This potent yet tasty sedative tea can be enjoyed by all ages, adjusting the dose as needed. You can take it as a daytime antianxiety tea, but it may make you sleepy. Using more lemon balm and less passionflower and skullcap will make it less sedating. The formula listed below is for a small cup of tea at just 4 to 6 ounces, so that you're not drinking too much liquid right before bedtime. You can premix a larger batch and keep it on hand. Double the herb portions if you prefer it even stronger. Feel free to add or swap in other infusion-friendly relaxing herbs such as chamomile, linden, holy basil, or a sprinkle of roses or lavender.

½ teaspoon lemon balm

½ teaspoon passionflower

½ teaspoon skullcap

½ teaspoon spearmint

1 heaping teaspoon honey (optional)

Combine the herbs. Pour 4 to 6 ounces of near-boiling water over the herbs and let steep, covered, for 15 to 20 minutes. Strain, then sweeten to taste with honey, if desired.

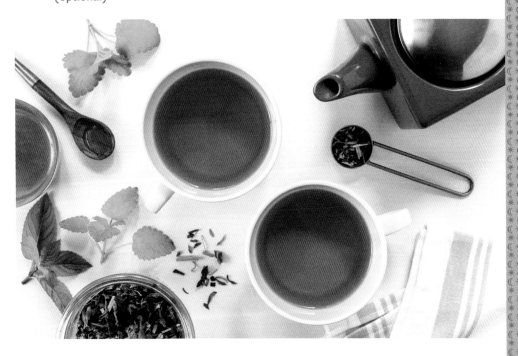

Holy Rose Water

Sometimes we need to take time to stop and sip the roses. The combination of roses and holy basil helps ease anxiety, grief, and stress while gladdening the heart and bringing joy to your day. This destressing drink couldn't be easier to make, and just gazing at your water bottle will gladden your heart!

1 or 2   fresh rose blossoms

2 or 3   holy basil sprigs

Combine the herbs in a clear glass container (for your viewing pleasure) and cover with water. Let sit in the fridge or at room temperature for a few hours before serving. The holy basil imparts flavor within minutes, but the roses take several hours to kick in. Drink it by the end of the day while it's still fresh. Holy basil and rose are a natural combination. You can try this duo in seltzer or as a tea, too.

OTHER HOLY BASIL BEVERAGES

Holy basil's fabulous flavor and nerve-soothing, stress-busting properties make it a favorite beverage herb. Use it dried in tea. Fresh sprigs (including those blossoms you trim off to encourage growth) can be steeped in hot water to serve hot or iced. Or for lighter yet still delightful infusions, use cold water or seltzer. One of the great joys of summer! Try holy basil solo or consider these delightful garden blends, combining approximately equal parts of herbs. If desired, add a slice of citrus, edible flowers, or a fresh herb sprig for garnish and additional flavor.

* Holy basil and lemon balm: calm energy, mood lift, antianxiety, great for workaholics to de-stress and before bedtime

* Holy basil and skullcap: more relaxing, anxiety easing

* Holy basil and peppermint: invigorate the mind, boost energy, lift spirits

* Holy basil and green tea: in the morning for a mellow energy boost; cognition, blood sugar, and inflammation support

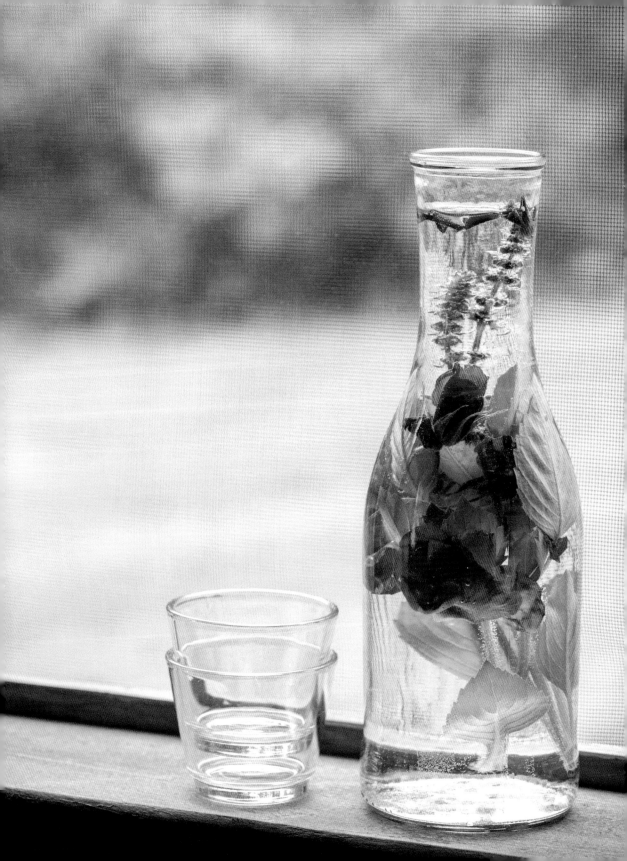

Happy Lemon Tea

Although I often combine lemon balm and holy basil, you can also enjoy lemon balm with other herbs and flavors. Its mild flavor blends well with more robust lemony notes, hibiscus, mint, roses, cinnamon, Korean licorice mint, and anise hyssop. Bland flavors like marshmallow leaf or root, nettle, or oat straw work well with lemon balm, too. Feel free to add skullcap or passionflower if you want to make it more relaxing. Here's a simple, tasty lemony blend that calms and uplifts, brightens the senses, and focuses the mind. (See the photo on page 121.)

2 heaping teaspoons lemon balm, freshly dried

1 heaping teaspoon lemongrass or lemon verbena, freshly dried (optional)

1 fresh lemon wedge

1 teaspoon honey (optional)

Combine the herbs. Squeeze and drop your lemon wedge into the cup. Pour 12 to 16 ounces of near-boiling water over the herbs and let steep, covered, for 15 to 20 minutes. Strain, then sweeten to taste with honey, if desired.

VARIATIONS

Lemon Cake Tea: If you add ¼ teaspoon of vanilla extract to this blend, it lends a lemon cake quality.

Happy Lemon Seltzer: Adapt this recipe to cold seltzer for a refreshing aromatic sipper. Combine 3 fresh lemon balm sprigs and 1 or 2 fresh or fresh-frozen lemongrass stalks into a carbonation-safe container (such as a reused soda bottle or swing-top beer bottle). Cover with plain seltzer and fasten the lid. Let infuse at least 30 minutes.

Add a lemon wedge and/or ¼ teaspoon vanilla extract, if desired. Best served cold or over ice. Add simple syrup or other sweetener, if desired, but it's delightful unsweetened.

Lemon Balm–Mint Tea or Seltzer: Mints also perk up lemon balm's flavor and work well fresh or dried, hot or cold. Combine lemon balm with spearmint, apple mint, or peppermint—each mint has its own vibe—or combine them all!

Sleep-Support Recipes and Remedies

Chamomile-Mint Tea

A simple chamomile or chamomile-mint tea is quite delightful, especially if it is brewed with good-quality herb for just a few minutes. Longer steeps will be more strongly relaxant but also more bitter tasting. This simple tea combo perks up the flavor of chamomile! Sip it with meals to ease nervous indigestion, relax, and support sleep. While any mint will do, spearmint blends particularly well with chamomile and may have its own sleep-supportive properties. Chances are you can find mint or chamomile tea anywhere you go in the world.

1 teaspoon dried chamomile blossoms

1 teaspoon spearmint or other mint of choice

Honey (optional)

Steep the herbs in 12 to 16 ounces of near-boiling water for 3 to 5 minutes (chamomile gets bitter if over-brewed; while helpful for digestion, most people find it unpalatable). Sweeten with honey to taste, if desired.

Tea bag tip: Chamomile tea bags are widely available and incredibly convenient but tend to be weaker potency than tea brewed with loose herbs. If you're in a pinch, go ahead and grab some bagged chamomile at a store or restaurant, but consider using two or three tea bags. Or combine one or two chamomile tea bags with one mint tea bag. Opt for organic brands, if available.

VARIATIONS

Try these variations, following the same brew tips as above.

* Catnip-Mint
* Simple Chamomile
* Chamomile–Lemon Balm

Tangy Vitality Tea

This recipe was created by Kristina Peebles of Climbing Vines Herbary and Colleen O'Bryant of Wild Roots Apothecary in one of my advanced tea-blending classes, and it's been a favorite of mine ever since. The primary goal of this tea is for calm, clear, focused energy and a cognitive boost. Schizandra is a cognition-enhancing, mood-elevating adaptogen that's mildly stimulating—especially in high doses or in sensitive people—yet also supports healthy sleep–wake cycles. Tangy red hibiscus brings the flavors together. It's quite sour and a bit tannic. A light steep is reminiscent of black tea with lemon, but a strong steep will benefit from honey or other sweetener to balance the tartness.

1 heaping teaspoon lemon balm, freshly dried

1 heaping teaspoon hibiscus

1 scant teaspoon schizandra berries

1 fresh lemon wedge

1 teaspoon honey (optional)

Combine the herbs. Squeeze and drop your lemon wedge into the cup. Pour 12 to 16 ounces of near-boiling water over the herbs and let steep for 5 to 15 minutes or longer. Strain, then sweeten to taste, if desired. (Consider brushing or rinsing your teeth after you drink it if you sip this regularly—the sour acidity and sweetener isn't great for tooth enamel. Sensitive tummies may also not agree with the acidity.)

VARIATIONS

Unrelated to sleep, I enjoy combining this tea with elderberry and sometimes ginger for immune support. The hibiscus makes this tea gorgeous bright red, but a sprinkle of butterfly blue pea flowers enhances the color and antioxidant profile even further. If schizandra berry is too stimulating for you, it's easily omitted, making these blends appropriate any time of day.

Sleep-Support Recipes and Remedies

Tart Cherry Soda

In studies, consuming a serving of tart cherry juice day and night on a regular basis can support sleep and melatonin levels. Tart cherry also has anti-inflammatory and detox-supportive properties, potentially reducing or preventing gout as well as exercise-induced pain. I particularly enjoy making this tasty, healthy soda/mocktail from the concentrate.

7 ounces plain or black cherry naturally flavored seltzer

1 ounce tart cherry juice concentrate, preferably organic

¼ teaspoon vanilla extract

1 lime wedge

Assemble in a cocktail glass, garnish with lime wedge, and enjoy as a posh, sleep-supporting beverage.

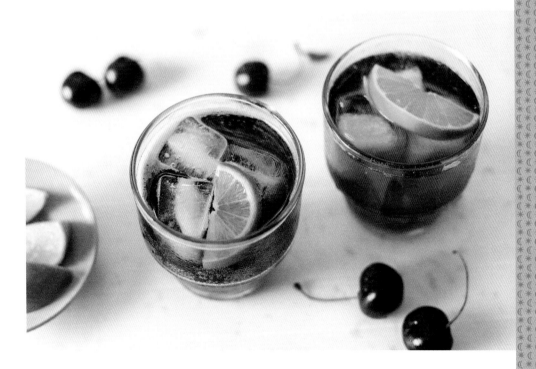

Lemon Bliss Seltzer

This tasty, refreshing drink combines the relaxing, uplifting, and focus-enhancing properties of lemon balm with the uplifting, delicious aroma and flavor of fresh lemon. The effects will kick in within just 15 to 60 minutes, and it's safe enough to sip all day or give to kids. Start with just 1 mL of lemon balm tincture—it might be more than enough to get you where you want to be. Increase if needed; some people might find higher doses too relaxing for daytime. Remember: Home-grown, recently made, fresh lemon balm tincture (directions on page 144) is vastly superior to store-bought.

6–8 ounces plain or lemon-flavored seltzer

1–3 mL lemon balm tincture

1 sliced lemon circle or wedge

Sweetener (optional; it doesn't really need it!)

¼ teaspoon vanilla extract for a more cakey vibe (optional)

Assemble in a cocktail glass and enjoy as a posh, bliss-inducing soda or cocktail alternative. Add edible flowers like heartsease pansy or calendula, if desired, for garnish.

SODA, SELTZER, AND MOCKTAIL VARIATIONS

Substitute lemon balm glycerite, vinegar, or oxymel for the tincture if you prefer it to be 100 percent alcohol-free.

In a pinch, you can combine 2 to 4 ounces of lemon balm tea with seltzer and lemon, but the flavor profile and potency will be different.

Skullcap, linden, chamomile, rose, milky oats, and/or holy basil extracts or teas are also palatable enough to sip in seltzer creations, especially with a wedge of citrus or other yummy flavor enhancer, like sprigs of lemon verbena, mint, or Korean licorice mint; fennel fronds; or sliced strawberries, lime, orange, or grapefruit. Fresh sprigs of meadowsweet, salad burnet, or violet leaf also add a surprising bright fresh flavor to seltzer or still water if allowed to steep for 30 to 60 minutes. Sweeten if desired.

Making a Tea Decoction

When we decoct herbs, we simmer them in water. This method works best for roots, bark, whole spices, and mushrooms, as well as herbs rich in minerals, polysaccharides, and carotenoids—basically tough plant parts and constituents that extract best with more heat over time. Again, feel free to play around with the exact quantity of plant material and how long you simmer it depending on how strong you like it.

1 heaping teaspoon to 1 heaping tablespoon dried herb

8–16 ounces water

Suggested tools: pot, hand strainer, mug

1. Place the herbs in the pot, bring to a boil, then reduce to a simmer.

2. Simmer for 20 minutes or to taste. (Decoct mushrooms for hours, even days.)

3. Strain and enjoy. Refrigerate extras and drink within 2 to 3 days.

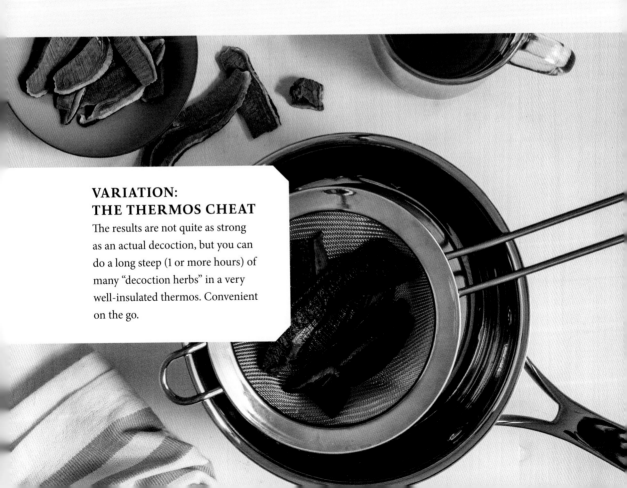

VARIATION: THE THERMOS CHEAT

The results are not quite as strong as an actual decoction, but you can do a long steep (1 or more hours) of many "decoction herbs" in a very well-insulated thermos. Convenient on the go.

Ashwagandha Chai

This recipe pairs my favorite naturally caffeine-free masala chai–inspired base with ashwagandha, which perks up the flavor of ashwagandha considerably. Crushing or grinding the cardamom and star anise will enhance their potency but isn't essential. I usually leave them whole.

2   cinnamon sticks or 1 teaspoon cinnamon chips

2   whole cardamom pods

5–7   whole cloves

1   star anise pod

1   teaspoon ashwagandha root

Sweetener and creamer/milk (optional)

Combine the herbs in a pot with 12 to 16 ounces of water. Simmer, covered, for 20 minutes. Strain, then add sweetener and creamer to taste, if desired, especially if the medicinal herbs are still too bitter for you. Alternatively, you can also do the thermos cheat method (see page 131) for a few hours or let the chai steep in a French press pot overnight.

VARIATIONS

Powder Power: Both the spices and the ashwagandha can be powdered and simply stirred into hot water, hot milk, or honey. Super easy! The powders won't dissolve; stirring frequently and drinking the powder will provide a stronger medicine boost. Commercial premade chai powder blends also exist, which you can add to other herb powders like ashwagandha.

Reishi Chai: Add 1 or 2 slices of reishi* in place of or alongside the ashwagandha. It's a tad bitter but tastes nice, especially if you add milk and your sweetener of choice.

Adaptogen Chai "Mule": Mix the cooled chai—*without* sweetener or creamer—50/50 with ginger ale or ginger beer as a mocktail. Just be mindful of the sugar content.

Try other medicinal chai-friendly ingredients: Maca, shatavari, marshmallow root, oat straw, nettle, turmeric, dandelion root, or burdock root. If you want a more energizing blend, add codonopsis roots to the ashwagandha.

Try additional flavorful chai ingredients: Add a spoonful of quick oats (it makes it a little creamy!), fresh or dried ginger, a pinch of licorice, a pinch of nutmeg, fennel seeds, and/or ¼ teaspoon vanilla extract.

*Note that the reishi fruiting body mushroom should be previously simmered or extracted, not consumed raw.

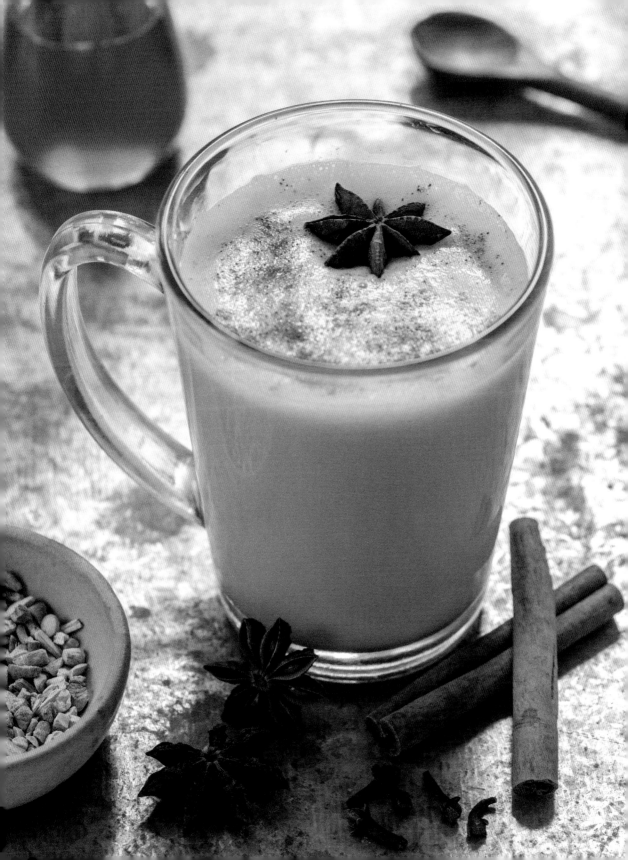

Adaptogen "Coffee"

Bitter and roasted roots make a nice caffeine-free coffee substitute. Adding adaptogens to the blend provides a morning boost with less overstimulation than you get with actual coffee. Be mindful that adaptogens and cacao may overstimulate some people, especially if sipped later in the day. If you have small intestinal bacterial overgrowth (SIBO) or simply aren't used to the prebiotic starches in dandelion, chicory, and burdock roots, you might get gassy with this tea. If it doesn't pass with a lower dose and a week for your microbiome to adjust, try a different recipe.

"COFFEE" BASE

- 1 heaping teaspoon roasted chicory root
- 1 scant teaspoon dandelion root
- 1 scant teaspoon burdock root

  Cacao nibs, carob powder, cinnamon chips or sticks, ginger, cardamom, or a pinch of nutmeg (optional, for flavor)

  Sweetener and creamer/milk (optional)

ADAPTOGEN OPTIONS

Choose one or a combination:
- 1 teaspoon ashwagandha root
- 1–2 reishi mushroom slices*
- 1 teaspoon maca powder

Combine the base herbs and any options, if using, in a pot with 12 to 16 ounces of water. Simmer, covered, for 20 minutes. Strain, then add sweetener and creamer to taste, if desired, especially if the medicinal herbs are still too bitter for you. (I particularly like blackstrap molasses, which adds coffeelike flavor and minerals.) Alternatively, you can do the thermos cheat method (see page 131) for a few hours or let the "coffee" steep in a French press pot overnight.

Note that the reishi fruiting body mushroom should be previously simmered or extracted, not consumed raw.

VARIATIONS

Mocktail option: Combine the cooled herbal adaptogen "coffee" (without creamer) with seltzer, ¼ teaspoon vanilla extract, and ginger beer or sweetener to taste. Be mindful that the sugar and adaptogens may overstimulate at night and the diuretic herbs may aggravate nighttime peeing.

Adaptogen Frozen Iced "Coffee": Make your tea an iced coffee via the methods on page 121; purée with ice and optional sweetener and creamer.

Using Powders

Although you can purchase herbs already dried and powdered, many commercial powdered herbs are low quality and easily adulterated. I usually prefer grinding my own. Start with thoroughly dried herbs. Grind well in a bullet-style grinder, coffee grinder, or blender. Some herbs grind more easily than others. For making capsules, it's okay if it's not perfectly powdered. But for incorporating into drinks or food recipes, it's best to sift the powder through a fine metal mesh strainer to get a more finely milled powder. You can sift it a second time through an even finer mesh strainer if you'd like. (Any large bits left behind can be made into tea or other recipes.) Store powdered herbs in tightly sealed glass containers in a cool, dark, dry spot.

WAYS TO ENJOY POWDERS

Powders are incredibly versatile! A typical dose is ¼ to 1 teaspoon, one to three times per day; see the individual plant profiles for specific recommendations on dose. Get additional powder and spice inspiration in Bevin Clare's book *Spice Apothecary* and Kathi Langelier's *Herbal Revolution*.

* Stir into honey; this is called an electuary. You can eat it by the spoonful. The honey helps preserve the powder longer, too.

* Mix into oatmeal, porridge, or chia seed pudding. Try ashwagandha and banana steel-cut oats with almonds, cinnamon, and nutmeg.

* Stir into hot milk (cow, coconut, almond, or oat) with optional honey, maple syrup, or other sweetener. Some nice combos include turmeric, ashwagandha or holy basil, and ginger; and ashwagandha, maca, or shatavari with cardamom and nutmeg.

* Make bonbons: Stir into nut or seed butter with honey, roll into balls, then roll the balls in toasted coconut or sesame seeds or dip in melted chocolate to enjoy as a snack. Good combos include holy basil and lemon balm; ashwagandha with cinnamon, cardamom, and nutmeg; and precooked reishi concentrate or extract powder with spices or chocolate.

* Add to smoothies.

* Mix into nut or seed butter.

* Blend with melted chocolate, dates, chopped nuts, seeds, and other ingredients to make herbal chocolate truffles, fudge, and other treats. Better for daytime remedies such as ashwagandha and reishi, but lavender is nice, too. Just remember that chocolate disrupts sleep for some.

* Add to hummus, bake into cookies . . . the possibilities are endless!

Aromatic Rose Powder

This delightful, earthy pink, and intensely aromatic powder can be sprinkled into coffee, tea, hot milk, oatmeal, golden milk, ashwagandha milk, shatavari, smoothies, chai, and the like. The aroma and flavor instantly perks up your senses and puts the nervous system at ease while also improving digestion. We crafted this recipe with Deanna Rose Sweeney alongside my advanced students, and it was an instant hit.

1	whole nutmeg	Grind into a powder in a bullet-style blender or coffee grinder. Store in a glass jar. Sprinkle approximately ⅛ teaspoon into drink, food, or other recipes.
20	whole cardamom pods	
½	ounce dried pink or red rose petals	

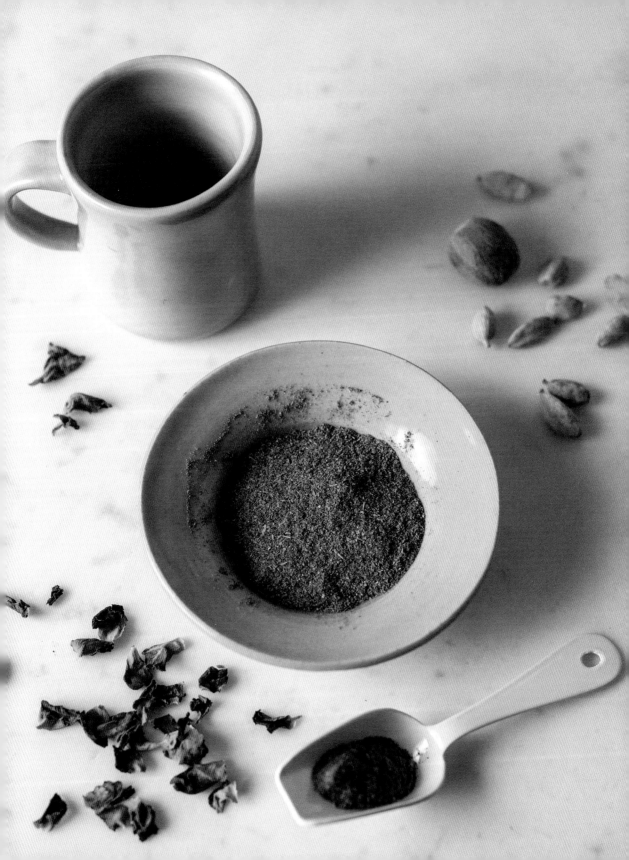

Warm Honey Milk
with Nutmeg

This isn't necessarily herbal, but I grew up with this old-time remedy. It's soothing and perfect on restless nights or if you wake up and can't fall back to sleep because you're feeling agitated or your tummy is irritated. Experts theorize that the honey helps release the tryptophan from the milk to relax the nervous system.

4–6 ounces cow's, oat, or almond milk

Pinch of ground nutmeg

1 teaspoon honey (optional)

Heat the milk on the stove or in the microwave. Stir in the nutmeg and honey to taste, if desired.

Sleep-Support Recipes and Remedies

Ashwagandha Golden Milk

Golden milk (also called haldi doodh) is a classic recipe from India and throughout the Middle East made with turmeric and hot milk as well as other spices such as ginger or a pinch of black pepper. I love crafting different combinations with flavorful and medicinal additions, ranging from spices like cinnamon, cardamom, or nutmeg to medicinal herbs like maca or shatavari, to powdered freeze-dried blueberries. Truth be told, ashwagandha isn't the best-tasting herb, but delivering it in a milk-based format is traditionally believed to help drive it to the nervous system. Combining it with turmeric also amplifies the anti-inflammatory properties of ashwagandha. The spices, milk, and sweetener enhance the flavor and action. But you could easily skip the turmeric and add whatever spices you like. I prefer to brew mine small and strong in an espresso mug, but you can use a teacup or regular-size mug if you prefer.

¼–½ teaspoon ashwagandha powder

¼–½ teaspoon turmeric powder

Pinch each of ground cardamom, nutmeg, black pepper (optional)

1–8 ounces hot milk (whole cow's milk or full-fat oat, coconut, or almond milk)

1 teaspoon honey or maple syrup (optional)

Stir the spices into the milk in a pot on the stove over gentle heat. Alternatively, microwave the milk, then stir in the powders. Add sweetener to taste, if desired.

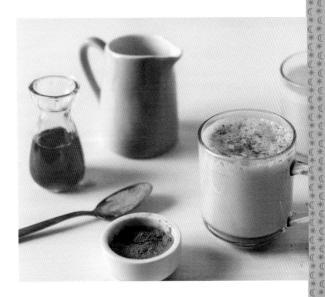

Capsules

You can easily make your own herb pills at home by putting powder into capsules. You'll get more bang for your buck with other powder techniques (below), teas, and tinctures, but capsules work well for convenience and herbs you just don't want to taste. If you plan to make a formula, measure your herbs by weight, then stir or grind them together so they're well mixed.

Ground herb

Empty capsules

Suggested tools: small, shallow bowl or
   capsule machine

Making Capsules by Hand

To make capsules by hand, place your powder in a small, shallow bowl. Pull apart an empty capsule. Scoop the powder into both sides, then snap the capsule shut. (Tedious for large quantities but easy if you just need a few.)

Making Capsules with a Machine

Make sure your capsule machine matches the size of your capsules ("0", "00", "000"). To use a capsule machine, load the machine with the empty halves of the capsules. Sprinkle the powder evenly over the side of the capsule machine with the larger capsule halves, using the scraper and tamper to push it over all of them and to push it down to get more in. Once the halves on that side of the machine are full (you don't fill the small capsule half when using a capsule machine), remove any extra herb powder, and follow the manufacturer directions to snap the capsules together.

Store filled capsules in a glass jar with a tight lid in a cool, dark, dry spot for up to 1 year.

Getting the right dosage. "00" capsules hold 300 to 500 mg of herb, which is the size I typically use. "0" holds less, "000" holds more. If you use a capsule machine, make sure the machine size matches your capsule size. But the exact amount of milligrams of herb per pill varies according to powder density and how tightly you pack the capsules. If you want to discern your exact dose, put a kitchen scale in "gram" mode, zero it out with 10 empty capsules, remove those, and then weigh 10 full capsules. Divide the grams by 10, and you'll have your approximate quantity of herb per pill (1 g = 1,000 mg).

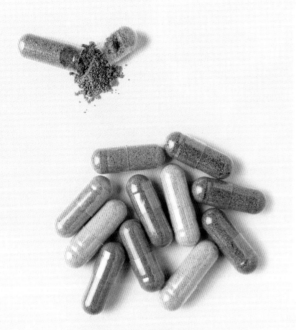

VARIATION: LOZENGES AND PASTILLES

No capsule machine needed! Great for "chill pills," bitter pastilles, and sore throat lozenges. Use your herb powders to make a dough/paste with honey/glycerine and water (add marshmallow root powder to help the mixture stick together, if needed). Roll it into a long, thin "log." Slice it into small pieces (roll into balls, if desired). Make sure they're a comfortable size to suck on or swallow. Dry in a dehydrator. If desired, sprinkle the pieces with herb powder or powdered sugar so they don't stick to each other. If you'd like to watch a demo, Rosalee de la Forêt has some great videos about making pastilles; search for them online.

Chill Pills and Powder-Friendly Herbs

These herbs work well (or well enough) dried and are good candidates to grind up for pills and powder creations.

- Ashwagandha
- Holy basil (freshly dried)
- Hops (freshly dried)
- Kava
- Magnolia

- Mimosa
- Reishi mycelium or heat-extracted fruiting bodies (not raw fruiting body)
- Passionflower
- Valerian

Tinctures

Every herb in this book works great as a tincture. It's often my preferred way to work with herbs that are more potent fresh (milky oat seed, lemon balm, valerian, hops, skullcap) or taste terrible. Tinctures are also convenient and fast acting, easy to keep at the bedside or in your purse.

A tincture is a liquid extract made with alcohol. Alcohol is as good as, and sometimes better than, water for extracting most plant constituents as liquid, and it makes a far more concentrated product. Instead of drinking a whole cup of tea, you take just ½ to 1 teaspoon of tincture. Dilute your tincture in a little bit of water (or whatever drink you like) when you take it because the high alcohol content can burn your mouth. Alcohol extracts have a long shelf life—5 to 10 years!—and they do a fine job preserving fresh plant properties that get lost in the drying process. They absorb rapidly into the body, bypassing digestion. (For a deeper discussion on tinctures and variations, charts and calculation worksheets, feel free to check out my website; see Resources, page 178.)

But, they *do* contain alcohol, which can be a problem for people who abstain due to a history of alcohol addiction or for religious reasons, or if they find alcohol irritating.

RELAXATION AND SLEEP TINCTURE SIMPLES

All of our sleepy-time herbs (valerian, California poppy, skullcap, passionflower, hops, lemon balm, milky oats, holy basil, motherwort) work well or even better than otherwise as solo tinctured herbs (called simples), and they can also be

Herbal Extracts

Technically the term "herbal extract" is vague and refers to an extract of an herb into a solvent of any sort—water, alcohol, vinegar, honey. Most often, though, *liquid herbal extract* refers to alcohol extracts, or tinctures. But if you prefer something alcohol-free, you can make extracts with glycerine, honey, vinegar, or any combination of them. *Standardized extracts*, often sold in pill form, are typically made with chemical solvents by herbal product companies to extract and deliver specific quantities of specific constituents per serving.

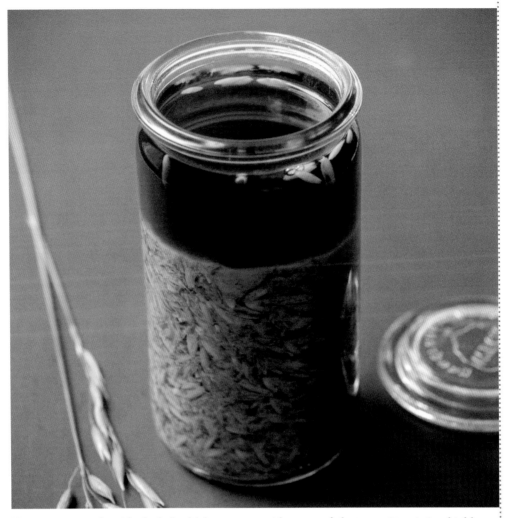

Tinctures are made with alcohol, which extracts a wide range of plant constituents in a highly bioavailable form with incredible shelf stability. It's one of our best ways to extract and preserve the properties of fresh plants.

blended together. Formulas tend to work well, though you might find one particular plant is the "it" herb for you. Dilute 1 to 4 mL in a little water to take just before you brush your teeth, and keep the bottle on your bedside in case you wake in the middle of the night and need another dose. All are best extracted fresh, though passionflower works fresh or dried.

Fresh Plant Tincture

If you have fresh plant material available, go with that for a tincture rather than using dried herbs. It's almost always better, and in some cases, it's really the only way to go. I love making fresh plant tinctures. With minimal preparation time, you're rewarded with a fantastic extract, and you fully experience your plant. High-proof alcohol sucks the water out of the plant and makes a better extract, but if you prefer to avoid it, see the note for alternatives. See the individual plant profiles for specific tips for each plant.

1 part by weight fresh herb

2 parts by volume 190-proof ethanol or vodka (or the highest proof you can get)

Suggested tools: scissors or clippers, scale, jar with tight lid, cloth, dark glass bottle

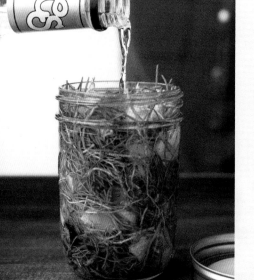

1. Coarsely chop your plant material with clippers or scissors. Weigh it out.

2. Shove the material into the jar—for leaves and flowers, squeeze in as much as is humanly possible.

3. Cover the plant material to the tippy top of the jar with alcohol (even if this comes out to *slightly* more or less than the 1:2 ratio—it's more important to keep it covered). You may need to hold the plant material down as you fill the jar and use a knife or chopsticks to remove air bubbles. Put on the lid. No need to shake. Open the jar a few days later to top off the contents with a little more alcohol.

4. After at least 1 month, strain the mixture through a cloth. Squeeze out as much extract as you can with your hands. A potato ricer, wheatgrass juicer, or hydraulic tincture press will also work well here.

5. Pour into a dark glass bottle and store in a cool, dark, dry spot. The tincture will keep for 3 to 10 years.

BEST USED FRESH
All plants in this book are acceptable as fresh plant tinctures, if you have fresh plant material available, but these are best used fresh: milky oat seed, lemon balm, motherwort, hops, holy basil, valerian, skullcap, and California poppy.

Dried Plant Tincture

I usually tincture dried plants when fresh ones aren't available; for example, if I buy rather than grow them. For most plants, fresh is preferred but dried will do. However, a few plants are actually best tinctured when dried. Many adaptogen roots, such as ashwagandha (shown here) are traditionally dried first to enhance potency.

1 part by weight dried herb

5 parts by volume 100-proof vodka*

Suggested tools: blender or mortar and pestle, scale, jar with tight lid, cloth, dark glass bottle

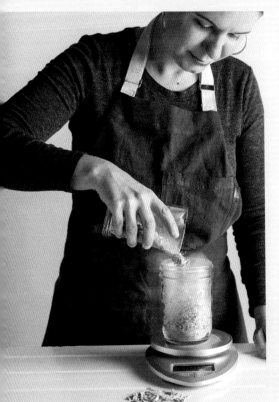

1. If desired, grind the herb coarsely in a blender or crush with a mortar and pestle. This improves extraction but is not absolutely necessary. Place the herb in the jar.

2. Cover the herb with alcohol. Put on the lid and shake well. Shake regularly, every day or so.

3. After at least 1 month, strain the liquid through a cloth. Squeeze out as much extract as you can with your hands. A potato ricer, wheatgrass juicer, or hydraulic tincture press will also work well here.

4. Pour into a dark glass bottle and store in a cool, dark, dry spot. The tincture will keep for 3 to 10 years.

*Vodka, preferably 100-proof (50% alcohol), works well for most dried plants, but 80-proof brandy or vodka (40%) works in a pinch. Or mix 6 parts 190-proof ethanol with 4 parts filtered or distilled water to get approximately 60% alcohol in your finished tincture. Use 10% food-grade vegetable glycerine with your alcohol for high-tannin plant material, such as barks, rose petals, or bacopa.

HERBS THAT ARE GOOD DRY

Any tincture in this book *could* be made with dry plant material if that's all you have, but plants that best retain their potency when dried include ashwagandha, kava, passionflower, lavender, cannabis, freshly dried holy basil, and mimosa. Most other herbs in this book are vastly superior fresh.

Maria's Go-To Sleep Tincture Blend

The combination possibilities for a sleep-support tincture blend are endless and easily adapted to the individual. Here's one of my favorite combinations. I typically make my tinctures individually and then combine as needed, but you could make a combo tincture from scratch if you prefer.

40% passionflower tincture

40% skullcap tincture

20% magnolia tincture

5 drops of flower essences of choice, such as valerian (optional)

Combine the tinctures and the flower essences, if using; shake to combine. Take 1 to 4 mL diluted in a little water before bedtime or in loading doses starting after dinner up until bedtime.

VARIATIONS

Potential additions or swap-out herbs include motherwort and lemon balm (these are my particular favorites!) and any other relaxing or sleep herb in this book. Vinegar, oxymel, or glycerite techniques could be used to create an alcohol-free variation; I'd suggest using dried herbs to reduce the risk of spoilage.

Relief Tincture Blend

In a pinch, a simple tincture of either kava or motherwort quickly calms when anxiety, panic, and tension have a grip on us. This blend is nice, too. I typically turn to the other recipes in this section for day-to-day use, but I'll recommend this blend for acute support as needed, day or night.

40% motherwort tincture

40% kava tincture

20% lemon balm tincture (optional)

5 drops of flower essences of choice, such as Rescue Remedy or lavender (optional)

Combine the tinctures and flower essences, if using, and shake. Take 1 to 4 mL diluted in a little water before bedtime or in loading doses starting after dinner up until bedtime.

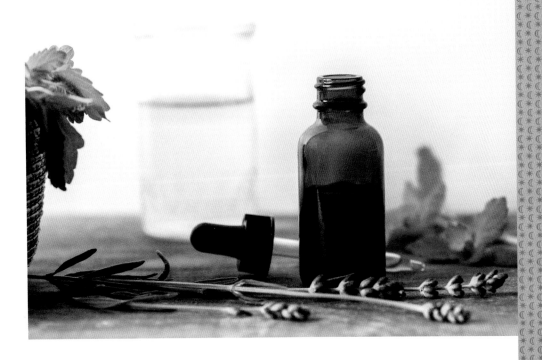

Stress Relief Tincture Blend

Herbalists and herb enthusiasts often make individual tinctures that they can blend into myriad formulas as needed. This avoids issues of combining plants that may have different extraction methods (and it gives you more versatility to change your formula as desired). For example, lemon balm and milky oat seed are extracted best fresh in high-proof alcohol, while my preferred method of extracting dried ashwagandha is in lower-proof alcohol. Here's one sample blend that has a mix of adaptogens and nervines to improve mood, stress resistance, and brain function. Use glycerites (see page 150) instead of tinctures if you prefer a sweet-tasting alcohol-free blend. Play around and make your own custom blends. To make the following recipe in a 2-ounce bottle, use 12 mL for the 20 percent ingredients and 24 mL for the ashwagandha.

40% ashwagandha tincture

20% holy basil tincture

20% milky oat seed tincture

20% lemon balm tincture

Suggested tools: Mini-measure shot glass or graduated cylinder, small funnel, 2-ounce dropper bottle

Measure each part by volume and pour it into your bottle. The dose for this blend would be 2 squirts (roughly 2 mL or ½ teaspoon) one to three times per day. If after 2 weeks you feel like you need a bigger boost, bump up to 4 or 5 squirts (1 teaspoon) one to two times per day. Dilute the tincture in a small glass of water or juice and take with food.

VARIATIONS

Less stimulating: If ashwagandha is too simulating for you, simply cut it out and use equal parts of the remaining three herbs. An equal part of magnolia or mimosa bark would also blend well and still support you day or night.

Even more relaxing: Add in skullcap, motherwort, and/or passionflower.

Make mine a glycerite: You can craft any of these blends as a glycerite using the maceration or simmered still glycerite methods.

Hops Citrus Nightcap Bitters

Herbalists adore digestive herbal bitters to simulate the juices and motility so that we better digest our food. This recipe is inspired by a batch of bitters I picked up in Maine that combined hops, pine, and other local ingredients. Add hops bitters to seltzer with dinner. In a pinch, you can simply use plain hops tincture or hops glycerite.

Fresh or freshly dried hops, coarsely chopped

Optional additions: fresh pine needles, juniper berries, ginger, coriander. Mild bitter-relaxing options include chamomile, lemon balm, or wood betony. Stronger bitter herbs include motherwort, blue vervain, and citrus peel or pith.

Freshly grated zest of 1 lemon, orange, or grapefruit

1 ounce fresh-squeezed lemon, orange, or grapefruit juice

100-, 151-, or 190-proof vodka or ethanol

Loosely pack an 8-ounce jar with hops (mix in other optional ingredients, if using), and add the zest and juice. Cover to the top with alcohol. Shake regularly and strain after 1 month. Add 1 to 3 mL to seltzer or bedtime mocktails. Serve with a wedge of lemon, orange, or grapefruit. Sweeten with simple syrup, honey, or fresh-squeezed and strained orange juice, if desired.

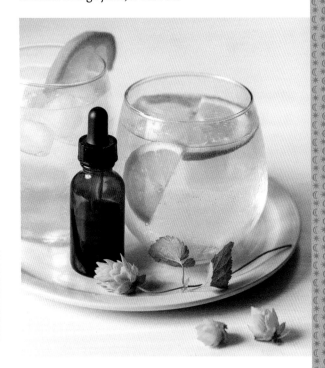

VARIATIONS

Lazy Bitters: Simply add hops tincture or glycerite to seltzer with a wedge of citrus.

Alcohol-free bitters: Use glycerine, vinegar, or a vinegar-honey combination instead of alcohol.

Herbal Glycerites

Sweet, sugar-free, and alcohol-free, glycerites are a popular substitute for alcohol extracts, particularly for children and recovering alcoholics. Glycerine soothes irritation and improves the flavor of blends, too. It keeps relatively well on the shelf. Glycerine does not kill germs like alcohol and vinegar do; it simply maintains the current germ status, preventing further or future microbial growth. Downsides? Food-grade glycerine costs more than alcohol, yet it's not as potent or shelf stable, and you need to take a bigger dose.

Great Glycerite Simples

Any herb in this book could be made into a glycerine extract, but the best options are aromatic herbs, those that maintain their potency once dried, and those with volatile compounds that must be captured immediately after drying. While certain "fresh" herbs listed below will be potent with fresh plants, they tend to have a much shorter shelf life. Some of your best glycerite options are as follows. Enjoy them solo. They blend well with each other in formula, too.

- Holy basil (fresh or freshly dried)
- Rose petals (fresh or freshly dried)
- Milky oat (best fresh, but it might get funky)
- Lemon balm (fresh, gently wilted, or freshly dried)
- Hops (freshly dried)
- Catnip (freshly dried)
- Chamomile (fresh or freshly dried)
- Lavender (fresh or freshly dried)
- Skullcap (fresh, gently wilted, or freshly dried)
- Motherwort (fresh, wilted, or freshly dried)

Making a Glycerite

I love this "sealed simmer" glycerite technique I learned from Thomas Easley and Steven Horne, which is done in a day. It's excellent for aromatic herbs.

1 part dried cut/sifted herb (*not* powdered) by weight or 2 parts chopped fresh by weight

5 parts glycerine by volume (70%/30% glycerine/ distilled water for dried plants, 100% glycerine for fresh)

Suggested tools: Large glass measuring cup, canning jar with canning lid, pot with lid that fits the jar, jar lifter, strainer, bottles—all sanitized

1. Cover the plant with glycerine (or glycerine/water), leaving approximately 1-inch headspace in the jar.

2. Screw on the canning lid. Place in the pot, cover completely with water, bring to a boil, then reduce to a simmer. Simmer for 15 minutes or longer.

3. Remove the jar from the water bath with the jar lifter.

4. Let the jar cool completely before straining into sanitized bottles. Best stored in the fridge, though they may keep at room temperature; in particular, glycerites made with dried herbs will have a longer shelf life. A well-made glycerite will keep for 1 year or longer.

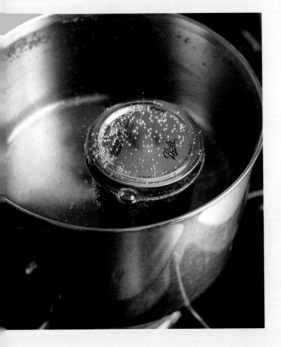

VARIATIONS

Macerated glycerite: Using the same ratios as above, fill your jar to the brim, shake regularly or keep the herbs submerged with a glass fermentation weight, and let it macerate as you would a tincture, straining after 2 to 4 weeks. Macerated rose petal glycerite is *delightful* (see page 152).

Glycerine transfer: If you'd like to remove the alcohol and water from a tincture to turn it into a glycerite, simmer equal parts (e.g., 1 ounce tincture plus 1 ounce glycerine) in a double boiler, uncovered, until all the water and alcohol have evaporated, leaving you with 1 ounce of glycerine extract in the pot. You will lose aromatics via this process but you may have a stronger extract of other constituents versus a standard glycerite.

Mellow Me Glycerite

Consider this blend as a daily tonic or when you just need to chill out but still function during the day. It has calming, mildly energizing, heart-gladdening, and cognition-enhancing properties. You can make it all together or combine separate glycerites together.

2 parts fresh holy basil flowers or aerial parts, chopped

2 parts fresh milky oat seeds, whole

2 parts fresh lemon balm aerial parts, chopped

1 part skullcap or passionflower aerial parts, chopped (optional, for added sedation)

1 part rose petals

100% vegetable glycerine

Follow the directions on page 151 for making a "sealed simmer" fresh glycerite. Store in the fridge. Take ½ to 1 teaspoon (3 to 5 squirts) twice daily or as needed. The shelf life of fresh plant glycerites can be unpredictable. Dried plants generally make superior, more shelf-stable glycerites; however, most of these herbs lose potency once dried.

VARIATION: TINCTURE IT

These herbs will be even more potent and have a better shelf life if tinctured, though the tincture won't be as yummy and sweet.

Lemon Balm–Catnip Glycerite

Carminative, digestive, gently calming, aromatic herbs extract relatively well in glycerine, especially in this "sealed simmer" technique that borrows from water-bath canning. Along with its sweet flavor, it's kid-friendly and alcohol-free. Watch for spoilage after a few months, if you're working with fresh herbs.

1   part fresh-wilted, chopped catnip or freshly dried

1   part fresh-wilted, chopped lemon balm or freshly dried

100% glycerine for fresh herbs or 70% glycerine with 30% distilled water for dried

Follow the instructions on page 151 for making a "sealed simmer" fresh glycerite, or combine previously made individual tinctures. Take ½ to 1 teaspoon as a dose. If using fresh herbs, store in the fridge or freezer.

VARIATIONS

Tincture: You can make this herb combination into a fresh tincture instead (directions on page 144), which will be shelf stable for years. Dose would be 1 to 2 mL.

Tincture/glycerite: Use a 50/50 mix of glycerine and 100-proof vodka for your extract.

Vinegar or oxymel: Use apple cider vinegar solo or mixed to taste with honey. The shelf life will be better if you work with dried or wilted herbs.

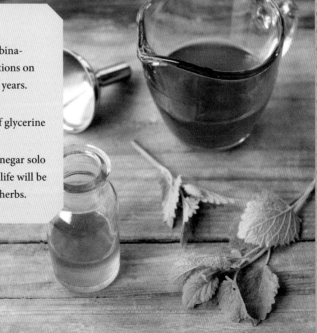

Flower Essences

Flower essences are made with a plant's flowers (even if a different part of the plant is typically used for medicine), harvested at their peak just as they're opening. They're primarily used for balancing psychosocial–spiritual states, though they can also affect physical conditions. Rescue Remedy is the most famous flower essence, a blend of five flowers used to bring calm in cases of trauma, anxiety, panic, and shock.

These highly dilute vibrational essences can be used in drop doses for emotional and psychological well-being (as well as spiritual and physical). They are very safe and are unlikely to interact with medications. Because they are extremely dilute, a little goes a long way, so they're also the most sustainable, low-impact way to make plant medicine. Blend them with herbal formulas or use them solo. Just a few drops on the tongue or in your drink will do. Bach and FES brands are the most common found in stores, but many small-scale herb companies also make flower essences and blends (see Resources, page 178); you can also make your own. Some of my favorites include the following.

* Rescue Remedy, a commercial blend by the Bach company of five essences, aids trauma, anxiety, and panic attack. The "Sleep" version adds white chestnut for swirling thoughts.

* Lavender (like the essential oil) delivers spiritual and emotional calm.

* Aspen quells deep fear.

* Valerian brings a state of deep peace and calm.

* St. John's wort brings light-filled protection from nightmares, dark thoughts, and hypersensitivity to others.

* Dandelion helps you relax and feel joy.

Ways to Work with Flower Essences

- Take 1 to 5 drops of the stock or dosage bottle on the tongue one to three times a day, or as needed.
- Add to your drinking water, tea, beverages, or animal water bowls.
- Add a few drops to tinctures, creams, salves, or aromatherapy sprays.
- Place a drop or two on the skin.

Sleep-Support Recipes and Remedies

Making a Flower Essence

Creating your own flower essences is a simple yet deeply meaningful experience, connecting you with the plants in a near-spiritual way. Approach it with the mindfulness you'd bring to meditation or prayer.

Fresh flowers

Water, distilled or filtered

Brandy

Suggested tools: scissors, small clear glass bowl or cup, small strainer, 4-ounce bottles with caps, funnel, ½-ounce dropper bottle

VARIATIONS

Homeopathic remedy: Homeopathic remedies are made in a similar fashion. In one method, you can start by making an herbal tincture as you normally would. Then dilute 9 drops of this in a 1-ounce bottle of 80-proof vodka. This is a 1 percent dilution or 1C. "C" stands for the Roman numeral 100, meaning it's diluted 1 to the 100th time. (To make 1X, or 10 percent—diluted 1 to the 10th time—dilute 3 mL in the 1-ounce bottle.) Shake vigorously between each dilution. Take 1 to 3 drops as a dose.

Low-dose tincture: Matthew Wood teaches us to use regular tinctures like flower essences or homeopathic remedies. Simply take 1 to 3 drops as needed. You could work with other types of herbal extracts similarly, too.

1. On a clear, sunny day without much wind, carefully harvest a few flowers from your desired plant, preferably in late morning. Place them in a glass bowl or cup filled with 2 ounces of water.

2. Place the glass in a sunny spot to sit for a few hours. The flowers float on top.

3. After a few hours have passed, bring the glass inside, strain the flowers, and fill your 4-ounce bottle halfway with the flower essence water. Fill the remaining half of the bottle with brandy (to preserve) and shake vigorously. This is your mother essence.

4. To make a stock bottle, fill a 4-ounce bottle 30 to 50 percent full with brandy, and top with water. Add 5 drops of mother essence. Shake vigorously. Use this stock bottle directly, add it to other recipes, or dilute it further into a dosage bottle.

5. To make a dosage bottle, fill a ½-ounce dropper bottle 30 to 50 percent full with brandy, and top with water. Add 3 to 5 drops each of stock essence of one to five different plants.

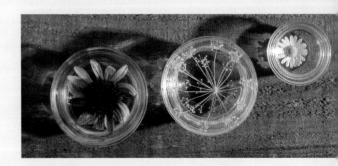

Aromatherapy

Essential oils may immediately come to mind when you see the word *aromatherapy*, but the art of plant aromas can be so much more than that. You attain the benefits of aromatherapy when you brush by an herb in your garden or rub and inhale a potted plant in your windowsill. Essential oils are *highly* concentrated aromatherapy extracts, and while they can be excellent, potent therapeutic healing agents, you can make effective, safer aromatherapy remedies in your own kitchen. It's not practical to make essential oils at home due to the equipment and humongous amount of plant material needed. Lavender, which produces essential oil easily, requires approximately *16 pounds* of buds (each pound is the size of a throw pillow) to make *1 ounce* of oil. Meanwhile, you need *1 ton* of rose petals to steam-distill 1 ounce, which is why true, pure rose essential oil runs $600 to $1,000 a bottle. So what can a home herbalist do? Plenty! Enjoy these tips, including several borrowed from the vivacious herbal aromatherapist Jessica LaBrie.

* **Steam.** Bring water to a boil, add herbs, remove from the heat, cover. Let steep for a few minutes. Then open the lid, lean over the water, and cover yourself with a towel. Make sure the water has cooled enough so that the steam won't burn your skin.

* **Hydrosol.** Hydrosols extract distilled water that contains a few drops of essential oil, making a lightly aromatic remedy that you can use in food and elixirs, for topical application, and for aromatherapy. Directions on page 160.

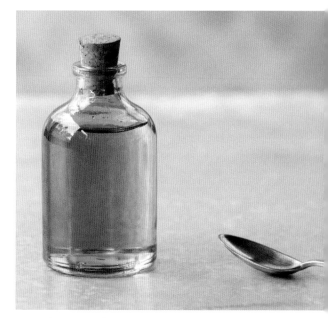

Rose glycerite is delicious by the spoonful, but you can also add it to creams for an uplifting yet calming rose-y aroma. Magenta seaside rugosa roses impart a delightful pink hue.

Sleep-Support Recipes and Remedies

* **Aromatic alcohol extracts.**
  Basically, you make a tincture (see page 144), with the goal of aromatherapy. Many aromatics extract nicely in alcohol. You can strain aromatic tinctures within a few hours to a day or two (as opposed to the usual month of maceration)—they often smell better with a short maceration. Use aromatic tinctures as sprays or perfumes, or add them to hydrosols to make them more shelf stable and add complexity to the aroma.

* **Glycerites.** Glycerine extracts (macerated or simmered still) do a lovely job capturing the aromatics of a plant, and you can use the glycerite internally or externally. Directions on page 151, rose glycerite on page 152. Holy basil makes a divine glycerite.

* **Tea, infused waters.** Drinking a cup of tea or infused waters provides aromatherapy inside and out! See pages 123–128 for recipes. Short shelf life, though.

* **Baths, soaks.** Aromatherapy while you relax! You'll absorb healing properties through your skin and inhale them simultaneously. Directions at right.

BEDTIME BATH BLENDS

Baths help deliver herbs' relaxing aromatics and other constituents to the body via the skin and inhalation. Great for kids and adults alike! You can make an herbal bath several different ways.

* Add ½ to 1 cup total dried herbs to a muslin cotton cloth bag, clean sock, or nylon. Let steep in the bath as it fills with hot water. Once the water has cooled to a safe and comfortable temp, step in. (You could also sprinkle the herbs loose in the bath, but it's a mess to clean and can clog your pipes if you don't strain the herbs out as your bath drains.)

* Brew a pot of super-strong tea using 2 ounces by weight of herbs in a half-gallon jar or pot, steeped 30 minutes or longer, then strain this into the tub.

* Dilute 4 drops of essential oil into 2 teaspoons of vegetable oil such as olive oil, and add to the bath. Note that this will make the tub *very* slippery—don't fall or use the shower until after you wash it out, or just make sure you're extra careful for the next shower or two! Skip the essential oils for kiddos. Also keep in mind that using undiluted essential oils can burn the skin.

Herbal Bath Options

Choose one or any combination of the following.

- Lavender buds
- Lemon balm
- Passionflower
- Skullcap

- Chamomile
- Holy basil
- Rose petals
- Spearmint (for added aroma)

HYDROSOLS

Hydrosols, also called flower waters, can be made from any plant material that retains its aromatics when simmered, which includes roses and mint-family herbs. Lavender and holy basil hydrosols smell amazing. A hydrosol contains distilled water and a small amount of essential oil from your plant material. You can make them with fresh (preferred) or good-quality dried herb. Hydrosols are technically shelf stable, but they have no preservative properties and often go bad after a few weeks or months. To improve the shelf life, store them in the fridge or freezer or add an aromatic tincture to bring it to 10 percent alcohol.

Great Hydrosols for Relaxation

- Holy basil (preferably fresh) is divine!
- Lavender (fresh or dried) comes out great.
- Rose petals (preferably fresh harvested in the morning) are nice but subtle.
- Lemon balm (fresh) will work but is iffy smelling.

Sleep-Support Recipes and Remedies

Herbal Sleep Pillow

It's fun to craft a little sleep pillow with dried herbs to tuck under your pillow at night and lull you to sleep. If you're crafty, you can sew your own fancy pillow. If not, simply use a large muslin cloth tea bag. Mugwort is a popular sleep pillow herb to stimulate more vivid dreams and help you remember them.

Lavender

Hops

Holy basil

Mugwort

1–3 drops of lavender or other relaxing essential oil (optional)

One large muslin cloth tea bag

Fill your bag with any combination of the dried herbs listed at left, plus the essential oil (if using). Tuck under your pillow. Refresh periodically, every few weeks or months, with new herbs and/or a few drops of essential oil.

VARIATIONS

Lavender in a pinch: Place 1 drop of lavender essential oil on a tissue or cloth and tuck under your pillow. Studies also show benefit for similar preparations reducing pain and anxiety in people headed into or coming out of surgery—a time when taking herbs internally is contraindicated.

Make a Hydrosol

This hydrosol recipe uses everyday kitchen equipment, but if you're *really* ambitious, you can buy a copper distillation still to make your own hydrosol and/or essential oil. Enjoy hydrosols internally, externally, in cooking, as a toner, in creams, and as aromatherapy sprays. Because hydrosols have a short shelf life, I often make an aromatic tincture (see Aromatic Tinctures, below) and add a bit to the finished hydrosol as a preservative—a trick I learned from herbalist Jessica LaBrie.

Distilled or filtered water

4+ cups fresh or dried plant material

Ice

Suggested tools: heat-safe bowl or large measuring cup, 1 gallon or larger pot with lid (no holes), canning jar lid or clean brick, metal mixing bowl, turkey baster or small ladle, 4- to 8-ounce bottle for finished hydrosol

1. Place your empty bowl or measuring cup in the middle of the pot surrounded by 2 to 3 inches of water. If your bowl is heavy enough not to float, place it on top of the outer circle of a mason jar lid. If it floats around, place it on a clean brick so it stays put in the middle.

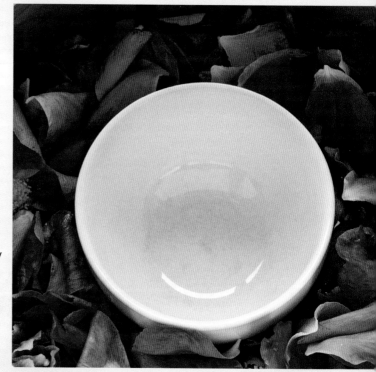

AROMATIC TINCTURES

An aromatic tincture is made similarly to a regular tincture, often with fresh herb (page 144). However, to maximize aromatic quality, we often strain it sooner—after a few hours to a few days—and it's okay if you use slightly less plant material.

Sleep-Support Recipes and Remedies

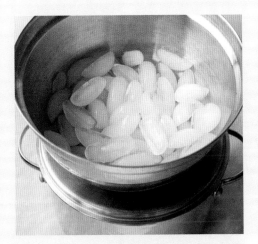

your aromatics). The steam contains distilled water plus plant aromatics. As it hits the cold lid, it condenses back into a liquid, drips down, and collects in the bowl/measuring cup.

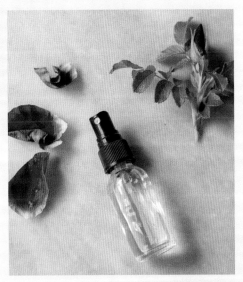

2. Outside your bowl, in the water, place your plant material. Put the lid on the pot upside down. Place ice on the top—you can put it right on the lid or fill a large metal mixing bowl with ice. The greater the surface area of ice on the lid, the better.

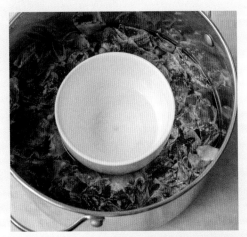

3. Gently bring the water to a simmer. Keep the heat high enough so that steam rises to the top but not to the point where the water reaches a roaring boil (which could degrade

4. Let this simmer for about 2 hours. Replace the ice/remove water from the top of the lid as needed (use a turkey baster or ladle if needed).

5. Remove the ice and lid. Gently remove the hydrosol from the bowl/measuring cup. You can scoop the liquid out of the bowl with a small ladle or turkey baster or *carefully* (with mitts or towels over your hands—it's hot!), without letting the plant material slip into the hydrosol, remove the bowl to pour out its contents. Hydrosols can go bad after a few weeks or months, because of the lack of pre-servative. If desired, combine with 25% aromatic tincture (page 142) to extend the shelf life. Or store extra hydrosol in the freezer.

CHAPTER 7

Herbal Safety and Quality Guidelines

Now that we've covered a tremendous amount of useful information on how, why, and which herbs benefit sleep, let's cover some common questions and important basics of herbal medicine. In this final chapter, we'll discuss herbal safety tips, special considerations for special populations (kids, pregnancy, and nursing), thoughts and cautions regarding combining these sleep-support herbs with medications or when transitioning from medications to herbs, tips for sourcing quality herbs, and how to best store your herbs. The information covered here will guide you to work with the best quality herbs in the most appropriate way, which will help ensure the herbs' efficacy and your safety.

Considerations for Special Populations

While the herbs in this book are generally safe for most people, no one herb is safe for everyone, and certain populations require special considerations. We have covered safety information related to herbal actions (such as adaptogen and sedative cautions) and in each individual plant profile. Tips for choosing and taking herbs appear on page 118, and guidance on when to see a doctor or holistic professional is on page 20. Here are some general safety tips as well as special considerations if you are taking medications, if you are pregnant or nursing, and for children.

SAFETY RULES FOR EVERYONE

Most of the sources you can go to for health and herb information—including this book—offer general information rather than specific, personalized advice for *you*. You'll need to do some digging to pick out the best options for self-treatment, or see a practitioner whose approach will take into account your particular health issues and constitution, any potential herb–drug interactions that could arise during your treatment, and so on. Before you begin taking therapeutic doses of an herb (or anything, really) on a regular basis, I recommend the following.

1. Do Your Research

Information about herbs is constantly evolving and varies across cultures, time, and the herbalist you're learning from. Before you begin taking an herb, research it in at least three good sources, whether in a class, online, or in print. Look for sources that come from the perspective of herbalists as well as those that are research-driven— folk use *and* science. Herbal practitioners generally offer a better understanding of the nuances of herbs and the ways that they can be used. Researchers (who may not actually use herbs themselves) are more likely to list every potential side effect and drug interaction under the sun while discrediting folk uses that haven't been researched. (Do we *need* a double-blind, placebo-controlled study to prove prunes are laxative?) Both perspectives are useful.

Science can help us better understand herbs; however, research on the use of herbs is very limited in scope. Scientists are notorious for using inadequate doses and treatment time frames, active placebos, poor or flawed study design, or uncommon extracts of the plants, and for having a vested interest in pro- or anti-herb outcomes. Well-designed studies also rarely test the crude, whole-plant medicine that most of us use, partly because such studies are harder to fund—there's no profit in finding out whether a whole plant that anyone can grow themselves is medicinally useful.

Relying on a mix of quality sources for your research gives you a broader understanding of a plant's actions and potential pitfalls. See the list in Resources, page 178, for some of my favorites to get you started.

2. Listen to Your Body

While you should do your research, also listen to your body to see if the herbs agree with you. A tea that makes some people feel absolutely vibrant may not resonate with others or may even subject them to a mild side effect like stomach upset. If an herb's side effect is mild, you may want to try taking it a couple times (perhaps with a meal?) to see if the symptoms pass or if perhaps they were unrelated to the herb. No matter how much science or folk wisdom is out there about a particular plant, ultimately only *your body* can tell you whether the herb is working for you.

3. Confirm the Plant's Identity

If you're harvesting your herbs from the wild or your garden to make medicine, be sure you've correctly identified the plant. Don't take *anything* for granted. Even if you grew the plant from seed or someone identified it for you, mistakes happen.

Keep a couple of comprehensive plant identification guides on hand. Field guides focused specifically on edible or medicinal plants aren't sufficient; their exclusion of plants not deemed edible or medicinal makes it difficult to guarantee the identity of the plant in front of you. The most effective identification guides are organized with botanical keys such as flower color and shape as well as leaf structure, and include a range of plants. I list some of my favorite resources and more tips for plant identification on my website; follow the "sleep-extras" web link in Resources, page 178.

Plants are best identified while they're in flower, and secondarily when in fruit or seed, so you may need to watch a plant for a full cycle before going back to harvest the following year.

It's important to develop good identification skills before you start harvesting plants from the wild. Though most plant misidentifications are benign (e.g., dead nettles for stinging nettle), some plants are mildly toxic and others are downright deadly (e.g., foxglove instead of mullein). Don't get overwhelmed, though—you don't need to know the identity of every plant in the universe, but you should know the one you're harvesting, as well as the deadly plants common to your area. And watch out for hitchhikers—errant leaves, stray bugs—in your harvesting basket.

WHAT IF I'M ON MEDICATIONS?

Herb–drug interactions are modestly rare but always possible, so you'll want to do your due diligence to avoid the risk of unpleasant or even life-threatening interactions. It's also natural to hope to switch from pharmaceuticals to herbal remedies—sometimes this works well, but not always. *Always* talk to your prescribing practitioner before adjusting or stopping your medications or adding herbs to your protocol. If you find that your medical team is unwilling to work with your holistic interests or that they don't seem to listen to and respect you, find a new doctor and pharmacy.

Adding herbs alongside medications: In addition to chatting with your doctor to at least keep them in the loop, you can ask your pharmacist if the herbs you hope to take are likely to interact with your medications. Typically, pharmacists have more training and access to databases than doctors do for herb–drug interactions; however, they can't generally tell you what to take. In addition, it can be extremely helpful to work with an herbalist or naturopathic doctor for guidance—they will be best able to recommend the herbs most suitable for you and typically have herb–drug interaction training as well. We also discuss some of

the common herb–drug interactions for herbs throughout this book.

Changing from medications to herbs: This is tricky! You will absolutely want your doctor's support and guidance on whether it's safe and appropriate to consider going off your medications, how best to wean down, and what to watch out for—which may include labs or symptoms. Meanwhile, I *highly recommend* having a naturopathic doctor or herbalist to support you with which herbs will be most helpful and how to safely add them in alongside and as you wean down on medications.

When I am working with a client and their prescribing practitioner, we usually find it most helpful to *first* add in medication-safe holistic approaches to help them feel more optimal and build a better safety net, then the doctor can advise on how to slooooowly wean down the medication while we add in additional herbs if and as needed to provide support, always keeping an eye on things to make sure that the person feels well throughout the transition.

Please, please, please do *not* take yourself off medications without guidance. Going cold turkey or weaning too quickly off medications may put you in extremely unpleasant and even life-threatening states. The risk depends on the medication, its withdrawal symptoms, and important roles it may be playing in your health. Sometimes medications are essential. In this case, it may be more appropriate to find herbs, diet, and lifestyle changes that you can safely add alongside the medications for better balance. For example, I have plenty of clients who feel most optimal with their antidepressant medication alongside herbs rather than without their medications. Or they may take other drugs—for heart health, thyroid, insulin, and the like—that are non-negotiable due to the life-sustaining roles the drugs play.

Always introduce new herbs slowly to ensure they agree with you and are not causing an herb–drug interaction. Observe your body carefully to ensure you feel well, including an even-keeled mood, not oversedated, and so forth.

Here are some key potential herb–drug concerns that pertain to this book's topic and the herbs in this book (this is not an exhaustive list but will hopefully provide some guidance in common questions and scenarios).

The safest holistic options alongside almost any medication include nutrition, exercise, nature time, deep breathing, meditation, flower essences, and inhaled aromatherapy. The milder nervines and gentle adaptogens also tend to be better tolerated. Seek more data on individual herb safety, though. Practitioner guidance is always helpful, too.

Serotonin-boosting herbs and supplements—such as St. John's wort, 5-HTP, tryptophan—generally should not be used alongside serotonin-boosting medications, *especially* if you're taking more than one serotonin-boosting drug. Examples of these drugs include most antidepressants, including selective serotonin reuptake inhibitors (SSRIs) such as Prozac, Zoloft, Lexapro, Paxil, and Celexa; serotonin and norepinephrine reuptake inhibitors (SNRIs) such as Cymbalta and Effexor; bupropion (Welbutrin), tricyclic antidepressants; MAOIs; various migraine medications, including triptans; many pain medications, including opioids and tramadol; lithium; recreational drugs including LSD, ecstasy, cocaine, and amphetamines; cough medications such as dextromethorphan; antinausea medications, including Zofran; and the HIV drug ritonavir. Serotonin syndrome symptoms include agitation, insomnia, racing heart, tremors, shivering, fever, seizures, and death. We don't have enough data to know if cannabis and mimosa pose a risk as well; though practitioners report that they *seem* safe.

Relaxing and especially sedating herbs may synergize the sedating effect of drugs, including not only antidepressants but also sleep, anxiety, pain, seizure, and blood pressure drugs, other medications, and alcohol. In extreme situations, this could worsen sleep apnea, cause you to fall asleep at the wheel while driving, decrease respiration, lower blood pressure, and reduce heart rate. Start with gentler herbs and always go slow, in a safe setting, listening carefully to your body.

St. John's wort interacts with more than half the medications on the market. Not only can it interact with drugs that boost serotonin, as mentioned previously, but it also affects various liver detoxification pathways including inducing CYP3A4, which can clear medications from your system too quickly, reducing their dose and effect. This can pose a dangerous risk with many medications, including cardiac drugs, hormones and birth control, antirejection drugs, and more.

Antidepressant drugs are one of the most challenging classes of drugs to wean off of, and the process should generally be done extremely slowly over months, with lots of additional holistic support and your doctor's guidance and supervision. Some people do best staying on their antidepressant medications, or at a lower dose, alongside medication-safe herbs and lifestyle approaches. I have met many people who deeply regretted the

mental health tailspin that ensued upon stopping their antidepressants. Be careful introducing any relaxing herb alongside an antidepressant as it may increase sedation, but the greatest risk is with sedatives, as discussed earlier. Also be mindful to avoid the serotonin-boosting herbs and supplements unless you're working with practitioners to slowly introduce them as medications are weaned down.

Antianxiety and sleep medications typically sedate the nervous system (some also boost serotonin) and may also be addictive with unpleasant withdrawal effects. Be mindful of the sedation cautions listed earlier and seek professional guidance. Herbs are often supportive; however, sleep medications can be particularly challenging because you're dealing not only with withdrawal symptoms but also the need to address the original underlying sleep issue.

Blood-thinning medications interact with many herbs that have blood-thinning or blood-clotting properties. Herbs in this book that *may* affect bleeding or these medications include reishi, melatonin, chamomile, gotu kola, ginseng, St. John's wort, and leafy greens including nettle and green tea. More typical cautions are for dong quai, vitamin E, ginger, garlic, Japanese knotweed/resveratrol, and many others.

Herbal Safety and Quality Guidelines

SAFETY IN PREGNANCY AND NURSING

Even though many herbs are likely safe while pregnant or breastfeeding, we have very little scientific data to guide us in the safe use of herbs during pregnancy and lactation. I turn to my colleagues who specialize in this field, including Aviva Romm (who has several informative books, blogs, and podcasts) and Camille Freeman (who has helpful lists freely available on her website). While the "safe" lists are somewhat short, many great relaxing herbs are on there. Chamomile, lemon balm, skullcap, rose, oats, and reishi are among the favorites. Also see the master chart on page 174 for a quick reference. Camille recommends limiting or avoiding herbs in the first trimester and always starting with low doses. Further research the herbs and don't hesitate to seek the guidance of a skilled herbal or naturopathic midwife or other practitioner who specializes in herbs for this population.

KID-FRIENDLY HERBALISM

Parents of kiddos will be happy to hear that many of the herbs and recipes in this book are kid-friendly. Favorites include chamomile, catnip, lemon balm, milky oat seed, skullcap, passionflower, and linden. See the master chart on page 174 for a quick reference. For infants, sticking to flower essences, infant massage, and homeopathic approaches is generally safest. Also keep in mind that you shouldn't give honey to children under the age of 1. My favorite books on herbs for children include those by Mary Bove and Aviva Romm. For aromatherapy, check out Erika Galentin's *The Family Guide to Aromatherapy*. Or seek the assistance of a naturopathic doctor or herbalist who specializes in pediatrics.

It's not always easy to reason with a child when it comes time to "take their medicine," especially if it tastes nasty or you have a really finicky or anxious kid. You have two basic approaches: (1) force it down to get it over with quickly, or (2) disguise it and improve palatability.

Having a powdered or finely cut/sifted herb offers many options for easy hiding, especially if it doesn't taste *really* disgusting. Depending on the flavor profile, mix it into oatmeal, applesauce, smoothies, eggs, honey, nut butter, honey nut-butter balls, and so on. A bit of powder holds more medicine than you'd think, too: 1 teaspoon equals approximately 10 capsules! Powder dose depends on the herb, and sometimes cut/sifted herb works just fine, too. Keep in mind that some herbs don't work as well once dried, such as milky oat seed and lemon balm. With teas and liquid extracts, like tinctures, syrups, vinegars, and glycerites, sometimes adding or using a sweet base like syrup or honey is all you need, but other times you need to get more creative. You can hide these as you would powders, but often mixing them in sweet drinks works best.

Adjusting the Dose

For most children, you'll want to reduce the dose. Use age and/or body weight as your guide. Clark's rule can work for children, dividing the dose down by body weight and assuming 150 pounds for the average adult:

Clark's rule: child/animal weight in pounds ÷ 150 × adult dose = child dose

With safe herbs, you have some wiggle room, and you may find that individuals do better with higher or lower doses. Use the chart below as a guide.

Estimating Dosages for Different Life Stages

LIFE STAGE	WEIGHT	ESTIMATED DOSE	TINCTURE DOSE	TEA DOSE
Adult	100–150+ lb.	Full	60 drops	1 cup
Teen	around 100 lb.	½ to full	30–60 drops	½–1 cup
Preteen	around 75 lb.	½	30 drops	½ cup
Elementary	around 50 lb.	¼	15 drops	¼ cup
Preschool	15–25 lb.	⅛	8–10 drops	1–2 tablespoons
Toddler	10–15 lb.	⅒	5–10 drops	2 teaspoons
Infant*	5–10 lb.	1/16	2–5 drops	½–1 teaspoon

*Generally speaking, the less you give infants, the better. Lean toward the gentlest remedies, such as homeopathics and flower essences, as well as the herbs with a long history of use for infants, like chamomile. Don't hesitate to seek professional supervision.

Herbal Safety and Quality Guidelines

Buying Herbs and Remedies

When it comes to purchased herbal products, not all are created equal. Well-made products will be more potent, effective, and sustainable and less apt to be adulterated.

FRESH-CUT HERBS AND POTTED PLANTS

Fresh plants often taste and work best, especially if you plan to make remedies with them. Look to local farms and online herb farms.

* Choose local, organic (or chemical-free) suppliers run by herbalists.

* Purchase plants that look happy, not wilted, brown or blackened, mushy, or moldy.

* Double-check the identity of plants with reliable field guides. Mistakes often happen.

* If you plan to plant the herb in your garden, ask or research what growing conditions it prefers and if the seedling needs to be "hardened off" before being planted outdoors.

* Use fresh-cut herbs as quickly as possible. If you must wait a few days, ask the supplier or research how best to keep them fresh in the meantime.

* For additional growing tips, seed, and seedling sources, see Resources, page 178, as well as the growing information in the individual plant profiles in this book.

DRIED BULK HERBS

Use bulk herbs for tea and spice blends and to make your own remedies. They're invaluable, inexpensive, and often more potent than prepackaged tea, but quality varies widely on the market. Look to local herb growers, herb shops, natural food stores, and quality online suppliers.

* Choose organic (or ethically wild-crafted) brands that specialize in medicinal plants.

* Use your senses to gauge quality: Even when dried, herbs should have bold colors and scents; they should not be brown, "dusty," or bland. Herbs are best stored out of direct light. Herbs with good "markers" for quality include calendula (bright yellow or orange), red clover (purple blossoms), nettle (verdant green), spearmint (strong Doublemint gum scent), cayenne (bold red-orange), and hawthorn whole berries (more burgundy than brown, minimal white cast). For online purchasing, try placing a small order first.

* Though powders are handy, they lose quality quickly and are easy to adulterate. Choose the closest to whole-plant form that is still convenient for your use.

* If you can, find out where the plants were grown and when they were harvested. Herbs grown in China (or bought/sold through China) are often adulterated and may not adhere to quality standards even if labeled as organic. Ask if/how the supplier tests for identity, quality, and contaminants.

HERBAL REMEDIES

The average consumer walking down an aisle stocked with herbal pills has no way of knowing all the production details that take place behind the scenes. Short of doing a lot of research and calling individual companies with a list of questions, the simplest approach will be to purchase from companies that are truly dedicated to quality and have an excellent reputation in the herbal/supplement community. Also see my list in Resources, page 178.

* Purchase from companies that specialize in herbal products and are run by herbalists. These will generally be of higher quality than mass-market herbal products. See Resources, page 178, for some of my personal favorite brands. Herb shops and co-ops often sell quality brands.

* Seek certified organic herbs and ingredients when possible. They're usually better quality and have a solid paper trail to reduce the likelihood of identity, adulteration, and unethical wildcrafting issues.

* Read the ingredients list (including any fine-print "inactive ingredients") to see what herbs or other ingredients are included. Beware of synthetic ingredients, artificial colors, artificial flavors, and preservatives.

LOCAL CONSIDERATIONS

Herbalism thrives in small-scale, grassroots circles, and many of the best herbal remedies are produced by hand in small batches. Unfortunately, small-scale, local product makers often struggle to comply with the FDA's regulations (which are geared toward large manufacturers but don't offer exemptions based on company size or sales). Even though the FDA believes *everyone* should be GMP-compliant, personally I recommend supporting small-scale suppliers regardless. Here are some questions to ask to ensure good-quality products:

* Where are the herbs grown, and how quickly are they processed after being harvested? Does the product maker grow them themselves or buy them elsewhere? If purchased, from where? If they harvest or dehydrate their own

herbs, what are their conditions to ensure quality and avoid contamination? With powders (which degrade in quality quickly), what's the typical timeline between when the herb was powdered and when you buy it, and how is it stored in the meantime?

* How does the herbalist ensure plant identity? Avoid adulteration? Are *all* ingredients listed on the product label? (They should be!) Is there a lot or batch number?

* Where are the finished remedies made? If they're made in a home kitchen, how does the herbalist ensure cleanliness? Can you visit the production space? (For personal privacy, they may not allow you to see the space, but it's nice if they do.)

* How long do they store their products? Is there a batch or lot number on the product that allows the producer to know when each product was made?

* How do they ensure prepared remedies are shelf stable? How long are the products expected to last after you buy them? This is of particular concern for low-alcohol extracts, body cream, herbal honey/syrup, and oils.

STORING YOUR HERBS AND REMEDIES

All herbs do best in a cool, dark, dry spot. Heat, light, oxygen, and moisture spoil or reduce the potency of almost any remedy. Shelf-stable remedies and dried herbs do best in a pantry or cabinet. If you store them out in the open for an extended period of time, use dark glass or opaque containers.

Long-term shelf stable: dry herbs, tinctures, vinegars, thick infused honeys, salves, cordials, capsules

Short-term shelf stable (a few months to 1 year): hydrosols, creams, topical oils; oxymels, glycerites, and syrups preserved with alcohol may last for a few months on the shelf but keep longer and maintain freshness better in the fridge

Best refrigerated: oxymels, glycerites, syrups, watery infused honey, culinary oils (1 week), herbal soda (1 day)

Consider freezing: fresh herbs (preferably vacuum-sealed) and any extra batches of cream, oil, salves, or syrups for later use

Properties of Sleep Herbs

HERBS	FAST ACTING	SLOW ACTING	ENER-GIZING	ADAPTOGEN OR ADAPTOGEN-LIKE	COGNITION-& FOCUS-ENHANCING	UPLIFTING
Ashwagandha	✓	✓	✓	✓	✓	✓
Bacopa		✓			✓	✓
Blue Vervain	✓	✓				
California Poppy	✓	✓				
Cannabis	✓			✓?		✓?
Catnip	✓	✓				
Chamomile	✓	✓				
Gotu Kola		✓		✓?	✓	
Holy Basil	✓	✓	(✓)	✓	✓	✓
Hops	✓	✓				
Kava	✓					
Lavender	✓	✓				
Lemon Balm	✓	✓			✓	✓
Linden	✓	✓				✓
Maca	✓	✓	✓	✓		✓
Magnolia	✓	✓		✓?		✓
Milky Oat Seed		✓				
Mimosa/Albizia	✓	✓				✓
Motherwort	✓	✓				✓
Passionflower	✓	✓				
Reishi		✓	(✓)	✓?	✓	
Roses	✓	✓				✓
Schisandra	✓	✓	✓		✓	✓
Shatavari		✓	(✓)	✓?		
Skullcap	✓	✓				
St. John's Wort		✓				✓
Valerian	✓	✓				
Wood Betony	✓	✓				✓

✓? Depends greatly on the person and/or the exact action/characteristic, could be debated • (✓) Subtle action •
X Not appropriate • X? Might not be appropriate (debated and/or varies depending on the person and situation)

Herbal Safety and Quality Guidelines

NERVINE (NERVOUS SYSTEM RESTORATIVE)	CALMING/RELAXING	GREAT AT BEDTIME	STRONGER SEDATING	KID-FRIENDLY	PREGNANCY-SAFE	NURSING-SAFE
✓	✓?	✓?		X?	(✓)	
✓	✓	(✓)		✓		✓
	✓	✓				
(✓)	✓	✓	✓	✓		
✓	✓	✓?	✓?	X		
✓	✓	✓		✓		(✓)
✓	✓	✓	✓?	✓	✓	✓
✓		(✓)		✓		✓
✓	✓	✓		✓		
		✓	✓	X		✓
	✓	✓		X		
	✓	✓	✓?	?	✓	✓
✓	✓	✓		✓	✓	✓
✓	✓	✓		✓		✓
✓	✓	✓				
✓	✓	(✓)		✓	✓	✓
✓	✓					
✓	✓	(✓)				✓
✓	✓	✓	✓	✓	✓	
✓	✓	✓		✓	✓	✓
✓	✓			✓	✓	✓
(✓)	(✓)				✓	✓
(✓)	(✓)	(✓)				✓
	✓	✓	✓?	✓	✓	✓
✓						(✓)
✓	✓	✓	✓	✓	✓	(✓)
✓	✓	✓				

Metric Conversion Tables

Unless you have finely calibrated measuring equipment, conversions between US and metric measurements will be somewhat inexact. It's important to convert the measurements for all of the ingredients in a recipe to maintain the same proportions as the original.

Weight

TO CONVERT	TO	MULTIPLY
ounces	grams	ounces by 28.35
pounds	grams	pounds by 453.5
pounds	kilograms	pounds by 0.45

US	METRIC
0.035 ounce	1 gram
¼ ounce	7 grams
½ ounce	14 grams
1 ounce	28 grams
1¼ ounces	35 grams
1½ ounces	40 grams
1¾ ounces	50 grams
2½ ounces	70 grams
3½ ounces	100 grams
4 ounces	113 grams
5 ounces	140 grams
8 ounces	228 grams
8¾ ounces	250 grams
10 ounces	280 grams
15 ounces	425 grams
16 ounces (1 pound)	454 grams

Temperature

TO CONVERT	TO	
Fahrenheit	Celsius	subtract 32 from Fahrenheit temperature, multiply by 5, then divide by 9

Volume

TO CONVERT	TO	MULTIPLY
teaspoons	milliliters	teaspoons by 4.93
tablespoons	milliliters	tablespoons by 14.79
fluid ounces	milliliters	fluid ounces by 29.57
cups	milliliters	cups by 236.59
cups	liters	cups by 0.24
pints	milliliters	pints by 473.18
pints	liters	pints by 0.473
quarts	milliliters	quarts by 946.36
quarts	liters	quarts by 0.946
gallons	liters	gallons by 3.785

US	METRIC
1 teaspoon	5 milliliters
1 tablespoon	15 milliliters
¼ cup	60 milliliters
½ cup	120 milliliters
1 cup	240 milliliters
1¼ cups	300 milliliters
1½ cups	355 milliliters
2 cups	480 milliliters
2½ cups	600 milliliters
3 cups	710 milliliters
4 cups (1 quart)	0.95 liter
4 quarts (1 gallon)	3.8 liters

Recommended Reading

As you dive into the world of herbalism and get to know the plants individually, these are some recommended resources for high-quality and in-depth information about plants.

Body into Balance: An Herbal Guide to Holistic Self-Care by Maria Noël Groves
This award-winning book is basically a foundational herb course encompassed in a beautifully laid out 300+-page full-color volume. It takes a body systems approach—how each body system works, how it gets out of balance, and how to work with herbs as well as diet and lifestyle to bring it back into balance. Similar in format to this book, it covers a much wider range of topics, including nutritious herbs, blood sugar balance, cardiovascular health, immune support, brain health, pain and inflammation management, digestion and detoxification, and more. The book is inspired by my Home Herbalist and Beyond the Home Herbalist course materials, and it's now a required or recommended textbook in herb schools across the world.

Grow Your Own Herbal Remedies: How to Create a Customized Herb Garden to Support Your Health & Well-Being by Maria Noël Groves
This book is geared toward beginner herbalists and herb gardeners and covers easy-to-grow medicinal herbs, arranged by body system and health goal, with recipes, recipe inspiration, and detailed plant profiles. If you enjoyed the plant profiles, growing information, and recipes in *Herbal Remedies for Sleep*, you'll love *Grow Your Own Herbal Remedies*! For a quick overview of the growing needs for all the plants in the book (plus a few others), seed and seedling sources, and more, check out the free mega grow chart at wintergreenbotanicals.com/sleep-extras.

Alchemy of Herbs: Transform Everyday Ingredients into Foods and Remedies That Heal by Rosalee de la Forêt
If you enjoy my approach to herbs, you'll also love the work of Rosalee! Rosalee's books and website feature in-depth, well-organized yet approachable and easy-to-read profiles on the plants that also incorporate herbal energetics, history, botany, modern science, and delicious recipes. Rosalee's free mailing list, podcast, and YouTube channel are sure to inspire, as is the "herbs" section of her website, herbalremediesadvice.org. Rosalee's first book, *Alchemy of Herbs*, focuses on common herbs in commerce and in the garden, organized by taste and energetics. Her second book, *Wild Remedies*, coauthored with Emily Han, explores wild medicinal plants while also providing important tips and exercises to connect you with the plants, place, and the ethics of sustainable wildcrafting.

The Essential Guide to Western Botanical Medicine by Christa Sinadinos
If you're ready to take your herbal learning to the next level, this herbal tome has lengthy, *incredibly* detailed and slightly advanced profiles on many of our common plants in Western herbal medicine. It's self-published and somewhat expensive, but worth it for those of you who enjoy herbal academia and want to have a thorough resource that dives deep into the plants themselves. Christa also includes recipes and nice extras in the back.

Adaptogens: Herbs for Strength, Stamina, and Stress Relief by David Winston and Steven Maimes
David is among the most influential herbalists in bringing an understanding and appreciation of the world's adaptogenic herbs to the Western and North American herbal communities. This book is easy to read and use, and features a deep discussion on the topic of adaptogens and adaptogenic herbs, with helpful profiles on the plants. The book also includes a discussion and profiles of nervines, brain-boosting nootropics, and nourishing tonics. The book features many of the plants covered in *Herbal Remedies for Sleep*—and more!—and you're sure to learn even more about each plant from David and Steven.

Hormone Intelligence: The Complete Guide to Calming Hormone Chaos and Restoring Your Body's Natural Blueprint for Well-Being by Aviva Romm
Aviva brings her expertise as an herbalist, midwife, and medical doctor to this deep dive into ovarian hormone balance, which includes sleep management alongside diet, lifestyle, toxin exposure, supplements, herbs, and more. If wonky estrogen and progesterone levels from menopause, PCOS, PMS, and related concerns are causing you discomfort and disrupting your sleep, consider Aviva's book. My book *Body into Balance* also covers similar terrain with a stronger herb focus, while *Hormone Intelligence* goes deeper into the science of the how and why of whole-life changes, with an action plan to support hormone balance.

Glucose Revolution: The Life-Changing Power of Balancing Your Blood Sugar and *The Glucose Goddess Method: The 4-Week Guide to Cutting Cravings, Getting Your Energy Back, and Feeling Amazing* by Jessie Inchauspé

As you may recall from page 12 of *Herbal Remedies for Sleep*, blood sugar dysregulation is both extremely common and one of the primary underlying culprits in sleep, energy, and mood difficulties. Jessie's books and her Instagram page, @glucosegoddess, provide easily understood and doable tips backed by science to support blood sugar balance through simple diet tweaks. You can also find a link to a great free podcast with Jessie introducing the key concepts of her books, as well as a blog article with additional podcasts by me on herbs and blood sugar support via wintergreenbotanicals.com/sleep-extras.

Resources

Helpful Websites

Wintergreen Botanicals
My website is loaded with free information about herbs under the "Learn More" tab, including seasonal wild Virtual Herb Walks, favorite recipes, many blog articles, and the ability to sign up for my free newsletter.

Visit the "sleep-extras" page for bonus goodies, more book and website recommendations for specific topics, and quick links to helpful resources mentioned in this book, including a free sleep webinar recording (use the discount code BETTERSLEEP), podcasts and online recipes on selected herbs mentioned in this book, tips for blood sugar support, deep breathing demo, plant identification tips, plus seed and seeding resources.
https://wintergreenbotanicals.com/sleep-extras

Memorial Sloan Kettering Cancer Center "About Herbs, Botanicals & Other Products"
This online resource is one of the best for summarizing the scientific information on medicinal plants in an even-keeled format useful for medical practitioners, herbalists, and everyday people, too. The exact website URL is long and complicated. You're better off Googling it and then saving the bookmark to refer to later.
https://mskcc.org/cancer-care/diagnosis
-treatment/symptom-management/integrative
-medicine/herbs

American Botanical Council
This nonprofit organization provides a wealth of information to the public about herbal medicine, reviews of scientific studies, profiles on plants, and more. Although many of the offerings require paid membership (different payment levels provide different levels of access), quite a bit is available for free. "Register" for the free mailing list to stay up to date on the latest herb news, studies, and more.
https://herbalgram.org

Historical Information
For historical information about herbs, check out Botanical.com and henriettes-herb.com, which provide easily searchable writings of old European and United States herbals from a century or more ago by Maud Grieve, King's American Dispensatory, and others. These are just a few of the fabulous resources available!

Favorite Sources for Herbs and Remedies

If you're not growing your own herbs, I highly recommend seeking out the high-quality organic growers in your area. They will generally have superior herbs and remedies, particularly freshly dried herbs. Here are some of my favorite mid-scale farms with online stores that ship within the United States. If you're looking for skullcap in particular, try Gaia Herbs, Herbalist & Alchemist, Zack Woods Herb Farm, and Oshala Farm.

Oshala Farm
https://oshalafarm.com

Foster Farm Botanicals
https://fosterfarmbotanicals.com

Zack Woods Herb Farm
https://zackwoodsherbs.com

Healing Spirits Herb Farm
https://healingspiritsherbfarm.com

Misty Meadows Herbal Center
https://mistymeadows.org

Avena Botanicals
https://avenabotanicals.com

Blessed Maine Herb Farm
https://blessed-maine-herb-farm.myshopify.com

Herbal Revolution
https://herbalrev.com

Bulk Suppliers

If it's not practical or possible to get what you want from a farm directly, these are some excellent bulk herb companies. However, on the international market, the quality can vary significantly from batch to batch, and herbs are more likely to be 1 to 3 years old when you order them.

   Mountain Rose Herbs, Pacific Botanicals, and Diaspora Co. are the suppliers I use most often. Other bulk suppliers that I turn to less often but are handy in a pinch and may be more easily available in your local shop include Oregon's Wild Harvest, Starwest Botanicals, and Frontier Co-op.

Mountain Rose Herbs
https://mountainroseherbs.com
Has excellent selection and identity controls.

Pacific Botanicals
https://pacificbotanicals.com
Grows many but not all of their herbs, which tend to be a step above in quality and freshness compared to other big bulk suppliers.

Diaspora Co.
https://diasporaco.com
Sells a small selection of exceptional single-sources Indian spices, including chai blends and a golden milk haldi doodh.

Smaller-Scale Suppliers

Smaller-scale herb shops selling online are perfect for buying small quantities of loose herbs and small-batch remedies—especially if you'd like to support small herbal businesses.

Maia Toll's Herbiary
https://herbiary.com

Meadowsweet Herbs
https://meadowsweet-herbs.com

The Herbal Scoop
https://theherbalscoop.com

Sacred Vibes Apothecary
https://sacredvibeshealing.com

Moon Mama Herbals
https://moonmamaherbals.com

Alchemy & Herbs
https://alchemyandherbs.com

Ready-Made Remedies

For ready-made remedies, again, purchasing direct from local farms and herb shops that make their own remedies often provides the freshest and best quality, but these widely available brands also have products of excellent quality. Look for them in your local natural foods store: Gaia Herbs, Herbalist & Alchemist, Traditional Medicinals, Urban Moonshine, Wise Woman Herbals, Oregon's Wild Harvest, Herb Pharm, Banyan Botanicals, Organic India, Megafood/Innate Response, Nature's Way, and New Chapter.

Flower Essences

Learn more about flower essences at bachflower.com, from *Flower Essence Repertory* by Patricia Kaminski and Richard Katz, and *Flower Power* by Anne McIntyre, and from local flower essence teachers.

Index

Page numbers in *italics* indicate photos; numbers in **bold** indicate charts.

Index

mint
    Chamomile-Mint Tea, 127
mocktail, 130, 134
    "Coffee," Adaptogen, 134
motherwort (*Leonurus cardiaca*), 64–66, *65*
    growing and harvesting, 66
    Relief Tincture Blend, 147, *147*
mugwort
    herbal sleep pillow, 159

N

nervines. *See also* kava; lemon balm; milky oat seed;
        mimosa; motherwort; skullcap
    about, 53
    additional, 73–77
    relaxing, 63
neuroendocrine system, 27, 51
nighttime urination, 18–19
nursing, pregnancy and, 169
nutmeg, 77
    Warm Honey Milk with Nutmeg, 138

O

optimism and gratitude, 50

P

pain, 17–18
passionflower (*Passiflora incarnata*), 93–95, *94*
    growing and harvesting, 95
    Tincture Blend, Maria's Go-To Sleep, 146
pastilles, 141
pills, herb, 140–41
plant identification, 165
potted plants, herbs and, 171
powders
    Aromatic Rose Powder, 136, *137*
    powder-friendly herbs, 141
    Powder Power, 132
    using, 135
pregnancy, nursing and, 169

Q

qi gong, yoga, or tai chi, 50

R

recipes, 117. *See also specific herb; specific product type*
    choosing, 118
    tips for taking herbs, 118–19
refrigerating herbs and remedies, 173

reishi (*Ganoderma* spp.), 33–35, 77
    growing and harvesting, 35
    Reishi Chai, 132
relaxation, 47
    beyond herbs, 51
    mind-body balance, 49–50
relief
    Relief Tincture Blend, 147
    Stress Relief Tincture Blend, 148
remedy/remedies, 117
    buying, 171–73
    herbal, 172
    homeopathic, 155
    storing, 173
    tips for taking herbs, 118–19
restless legs syndrome (RLS), 19–20
roots, harvesting, 110–11, *111*
roses (*Rosa* spp.), 74, *74*
    blossoms/petals, 63, *63*
    Holy Rose Water, 124, *125*
    Powder, Aromatic Rose, 136, *137*

S

safety, 163–170
    Clark's rule, 170
    dosages, life stages and, **170**
    medications and, 166–68
    pregnancy, nursing and, 169
    relaxing/sedating herbs and, 167–68
    special populations and, 164–179
schizandra (*Schisandra chinensis*), 44–45, *44*, 77
    nighttime urination and, 18
sedating sleep support, 79. *See also* California poppy;
        chamomile; hops; lavender; passionflower;
        valerian
    dosing tips, bedtime, 82
    gentle sedatives, 82
    sedative herbs, 80
    sleep remedies, additional, 102–5
    stronger sleep aids, 92
    tips on getting sleep, 80
sedatives, 47
    importance of, 48–49
Seltzer, Lemon Bliss, 130
serotonin boosters, 103
serotonin-boosting herbs and supplements, 167
shatavari (*Asparagus racemosus*), 43, *43*, 77
shelf-stable herbs and remedies, 173
simples
    glycerite, 150

Index